Antiepileptic Drugs

Antiepileptic Drugs

Editors

Arun Garg DM
Director
Institute of Neurosciences
Medanta – The Medicity
Gurugram, Haryana, India

Atma Ram Bansal DM
Senior Consultant
Institute of Neurosciences
Medanta – The Medicity
Gurugram, Haryana, India

Foreword
Kurupath Radhakrishnan

JAYPEE
JAYPEE BROTHERS MEDICAL PUBLISHERS
The Health Sciences Publisher
New Delhi | London

Jaypee Brothers Medical Publishers (P) Ltd

Headquarters
EMCA House
23/23-B, Ansari Road, Daryaganj
New Delhi 110 002, India
Landline: +91-11-23272143, +91-11-23272703
+91-11-23282021, +91-11-23245672
E-mail: jaypee@jaypeebrothers.com

Corporate Office
4838/24, Ansari Road, Daryaganj
New Delhi 110 002, India
Phone: +91-11-43574357
Fax: +91-11-43574314
E-mail: jaypee@jaypeebrothers.com

Overseas Office
J.P. Medical Ltd.
83, Victoria Street, London
SW1H 0HW (UK)
Phone: +44 20 3170 8910
E-mail: info@jpmedpub.com

EU GPSR Authorised Representative
Logos Europe, 9 rue Nicolas Poussin
17000, La Rochelle, France
Phone: +33 (0) 6 67 93 73 78
E-mail: contact@logoseurope.eu

Website: www.jaypeebrothers.com
Website: www.jaypeedigital.com

Antiepileptic Drugs / Arun Garg, Atma Ram Bansal

First Edition: 2020

Reprint: **2025**

ISBN: 978-93-88958-24-0

Printed in India

Dedicated to

Our neurology team especially
Rajeev Goyal,
Susant Bhuyan,
and
Abdul Muniem

FOREWORD

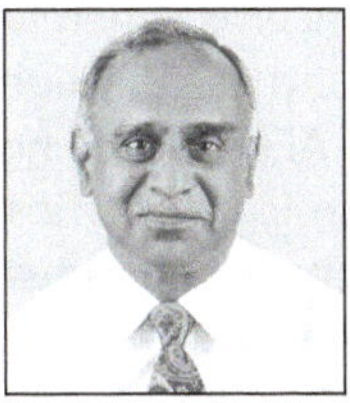

Kurupath Radhakrishnan MD DM FAMS FAAN FANA
Senior Consultant
Department of Neurosciences
Avitis Institute of Medical Sciences
Nemmara, Palakkad, Kerala, India

Former
Director, Department of Neurology and Head
R Madhavan Nayar Center for Comprehensive Epilepsy Care
Sree Chitra Tirunal Institute of Medical Sciences and Technology
Trivandrum, Kerala, India

Head of Department of Neurology, Kasturba Medical College, Manipal Academy of Higher Education
Manipal, Karnataka, India

Professor, Department of Neurology, and Head
Amrita Advanced Epilepsy Center
Amrita Institute of Medical Sciences
Cochin, Kerala, India

After making a fairly convincing diagnosis of epileptic seizures, patients are usually initiated on therapy with drugs to control the seizures. Although these drugs help in achieving seizure control in majority of people with epilepsy (PWE) and are therefore very effective antiseizure drugs, there is little evidence to indicate that these drugs influence the process of epileptogenesis [and are therefore truly not antiepileptic drugs (AEDs)]. However, by frequent and prolonged usage, the term "Antiepileptic Drugs", which the editors have chosen as the title of the book, has become so firmly engraved that it is very difficult to replace it by the more appropriate term "Antiseizure Drugs".

Over the last three decades, several AEDs have been approved and available for use the world over. Out of the more than 20 AEDs approved, a dozen of them are in common usage today. Although this scenario has made the choice of the AEDs more wide-ranging and evidence-based, it has resulted in widespread misuse of them especially in the developing countries, where majority of PWE are diagnosed and treated by the primary and secondary care physicians who are oblivious of the recent advances in AED therapy.

If correctly chosen and administered, AEDs can result in controlling the seizures in more than two-thirds of PWE. In those who become free of seizures, the AEDs can be tapered and successfully discontinued in the majority in due course of time. However, disappointingly, even today, more than half of the PWE in the community, especially in developing countries, do not receive adequate AED therapy or receive no AED therapy at all. The AEDs not being available and affordable, inability of the primary and secondary care physicians to choose the appropriate AEDs with respect to the type of seizures and epilepsies, myths and misconceptions associated with epilepsy contribute to the treatment gap.

Dr Atma Ram Bansal and Dr Arun Garg have designed this book to address the above-described concerns inherent with the treatment of PWE in developing countries. Through 14 chapters, the book covers every aspect of AEDs including history, pharmacokinetic and pharmacodynamic properties, choice with respect to seizure types and epilepsy syndromes, adverse effects, when to initiate AEDs, and when and how to discontinue them. Additionally, special situations such as AED therapy in status epilepticus and in systemic disorders, in women of the child bearing age and during pregnancy and lactation, and in children and elderly are also deliberated. The authors of each chapter have narrated the topics assigned to them in a comprehensive manner. Several tables and figures strengthen and streamline the text.

Although the editors have primarily intended the book for non-neurologists engaged in treating PWE such as primary and secondary care physicians, pediatricians and psychiatrists, postgraduate students in internal medicine, pediatrics, psychiatry and neurology, and neurologists (both junior and senior, who are not hardcore epileptologists) will also immensely benefit by reading this book. Let me congratulate the authors of individual chapters for the contributions, and the editors for elegantly compiling the chapters. I strongly recommend this book to each and every one involved in the treatment of PWE.

CONTRIBUTORS

EDITORS

Arun Garg DM
Director
Institute of Neurosciences
Medanta – The Medicity
Gurugram, Haryana, India

Atma Ram Bansal DM
Senior Consultant
Institute of Neurosciences
Medanta – The Medicity
Gurugram, Haryana, India

CONTRIBUTING AUTHORS

Aniruddha Vasant More DM
Post-Doctoral Fellow in Epilepsy
Department of Neurosciences
Medanta – The Medicity
Gurugram, Haryana, India

Ashish Bagdi MBBS MD DM
Consultant Neurologist
Department of Neurology
Convenient Hospitals Ltd
Indore, Madhya Pradesh, India

Ashok Panagariya MBBS MD DM FRCP
Ex Vice Chancellor Rajasthan Medical University
Ex Principal SMS Medical College
Jaipur Rajasthan
Consultant Neurologist
Jaipur, Rajasthan, India

Bindu Menon MD DM DNB PGDCN FRCP MNAMS FICP
Professor and Head of Department
Department of Neurology
Apollo Speciality Hospitals
Nellore, Andhra Pradesh, India

Dinesh Nayak MD DM
Department of Neurology
Director
Department of Neurology
Gleneagles Global Health City
Chennai, Tamil Nadu, India

Karan M Desai DM
Senior Resident
Department of Neurology
King Edward Memorial Hospital and Seth Gordhandas Sunderdas Medical College
Mumbai, Maharashtra, India

Neeraj N Baheti MD DNB DM
Consultant Neurologist and Epileptologist, Dr GM Taori
Central India Institute Of Medical Sciences (CIIMS) Hospital
Nagpur, Maharashtra, India

Sangeeta H Ravat DM
Professor and Head of Department
Department of Neurology
King Edward Memorial Hospital and Seth Gordhandas Sunderdas Medical College
Mumbai, Maharashtra, India

Shyam K Jaiswal MD DNB
Consultant Neurologist
Epileptologist, CARE Hospitals
CARE Outpatient Centre
Hyderabad, Telangana, India

Sita Jayalakshmi DM
Consultant Neurologist
Department of Neurology
Krishna Institute of Medical Sciences
Secunderabad, Telangana, India

Sudhindra Vooturi Master in Physiotherapy PhD Scholar Neuro-Physiology and Physiotherapy
Chief of Lifestyle and Rehabilitation
Department of Neurology
Krishna Institute of Medical Sciences
Secunderabad, Telangana, India

Sujit Abajirao Jagtap MD DM
Assistant Professor
Department of Neurology
Bharati Vidyapeeth Medical College
Pune, Maharashtra, India

Suresh Babu Pasangulapati
MD DM Post-Doctoral Fellowship (EEG)
Consultant Neurologist
Department of Neurology
Krishna Institute of Medical Sciences
Secunderabad, Telangana, India

Vivek Mathew MBBS MD DM DNB
Professor of Neurology
Department of Neurological Sciences
Christian Medical College
Vellore, Tamil Nadu, India

Yeeshu S Sudan MBBS MD
Consultant
Department of Paediatrics
Medanta – The Medicity Hospital
Gurugram, Haryana, India

PREFACE

Epilepsy is a well-researched topic with numerous books, monographs, and papers. The numerous literature also shows that there is lot of knowledge that we have acquired, however, lacunae still exist. The effort of this book is to package the best of current knowledge and practices into forming an individualized treatment algorithm. It also covers the diagnostic dilemmas, the myths and misconceptions regarding the disease, and the pros and cons of the antiepileptic drugs (AEDs) in achieving seizure control. The book has contributions from practical wisdom of epilepsy experts. It is a must-have book for any clinician involved in the treatment of epilepsy.

Arun Garg
Atma Ram Bansal

CONTENTS

1

CHAPTER

Historical Aspects of Antiepileptic Drugs

Aniruddha Vasant More, Arun Garg

INTRODUCTION

Today we have many agents with us to treat epilepsy. However, the story of how these agents were discovered is very interesting and fascinating. Many agents were not originally intended to be used as antiepileptics and their antiepileptic properties were accidentally discovered.

BROMIDE: FIRST AED EVER USED

The story begins in the 18th century and the credit of being the first antiepileptic drug (AED) used for treating epilepsy goes to bromide (Table 1 and Fig. 1).

TABLE 1: Antiepileptic drugs and their year of discovery.

Antiepileptic drug	Approximate year of discovery of antiepileptic properties/FDA approval for treatment
Bromide	1857
Phenobarbitone	1912
Phenytoin	1938
Ethosuximide	1958
Carbamazepine	1965
Diazepam	1965
Valproate	1967
Zonisamide	1989
Gabapentin	1993
Felbamate	1993
Lamotrigine	1994
Topiramate	1996
Tiagabine	1997
Levetiracetam	1999
Oxcarbazepine	2000
Pregabalin	2005
Rufinamide	2007
Lacosamide	2008
Eslicarbazepine	2009
Perampanel	2012

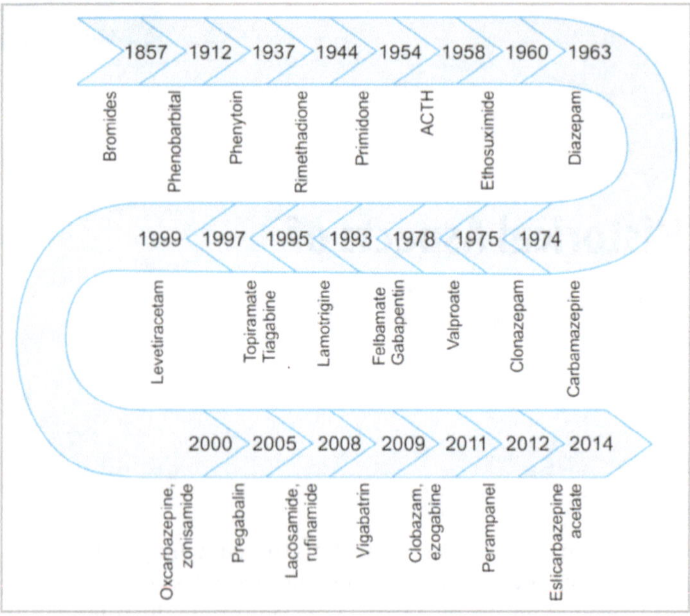

FIG. 1: Antiepileptic drugs and their year of discovery.

On May 11, 1857, Sir Charles Lacock, who was Queen Victoria's personal physician, first mentioned the use of bromide for treating epilepsy at a meeting of the Royal Medical and Chirurgical Society held in London.[1] He had successfully treated a female suffering from so-called "hysterical epilepsy" using bromide. In that era, epilepsy was attributed to uterine irritation, sexual excitement and menstruation (hence the term hysterical epilepsy; hysteros = uterus). Probably the patient Lacock had treated and other subjects with so-called "hysterical epilepsy" might have had catamenial epilepsy. Why Lacock thought of using bromide in epilepsy? Because he had read a German report, which stated that bromide caused reversible sexual impotence prompting him to use it in the female suffering from epilepsy to calm down her sexual excitement/uterine irritation.[1] However, Lacock did not publish his experience about the efficacy of bromides until Dr Charles Bland Radcliffe credited him with the discovery of bromides in 1860 based on his personal experience of the use of bromides in effectively controlling epilepsy. Gradually, bromide became a popular agent for treating epilepsy and remained so for many years. However, its use was associated with bromism, which manifested with dermatological conditions such as severe rash and psychological symptoms such as irritability, emotional instability, schizophrenia-like psychosis, memory disturbance and dementia. This led to a gradual decline in the popularity of bromide.[2] The subsequent emergence of phenobarbitone as a safe and effective AED led to the almost complete demise of this drug.

ACCIDENTAL DISCOVERY OF PHENOBARBITONE

The antiepileptic properties of phenobarbitone were accidentally discovered by Alfred Hauptmann, a German psychiatrist in the year 1912. Before its antiepileptic properties were discovered, phenobarbitone (then branded as Luminal) was used as a hypnotic/sedative drug, which was marketed by F. Bayer and Company. Hauptmann in his residency days used to stay near a ward full of epilepsy patients. He was particularly troubled by patients having seizures at night because of which they kept falling out of bed. To have a sound sleep at night, he once gave phenobarbitone to his patients with an intention to sedate them. Not only did he sleep well that night but to his surprise patients who were given phenobarbitone did not have seizures next day leading him to publish his findings and thus highlighting antiepileptic properties of this drug.[3] To commemorate his landmark contribution in the field of epilepsy, the Alfred-Hauptmann Award is given for epilepsy research. Phenobarbitone after its discovery continued to remain a popular and effective AED even till date. However, sedative properties of phenobarbitone prompted a need for the search of a less sedative but equally effective AED, which led to the discovery of phenytoin in the year 1938.

THE ERA OF CONVENTIONAL AEDS

Tracy Putnam, the director of neurology unit in Boston city hospital wanted to try out nonsedative phenyl compounds provided to him by Parke, Davis and Company. Phenytoin was the only safe compound amongst them. It was found that phenytoin was very effective in preventing electrically induced convulsions in cats. So, Putnam gave it to one of his assistant Houston Merritt for clinical use. He found out that it effectively controlled seizures in a patient who had suffered seizures for many years thus bringing it in routine practice as an effective AED without any sedative effects.[4] Next anticonvulsant to be discovered was carbamazepine by a chemist Walter Schindler at JR Geigy Ltd (now Novartis), Switzerland, in 1953. He developed this tricyclic compound along with imipramine when he was trying to find alternatives for chlorpromazine.[4] However, it was not first marketed as an AED but as a medication for trigeminal neuralgia in the year 1962. One year later, its anticonvulsive properties were confirmed by randomized trials and it was marketed in Europe for epilepsy in 1965. However, its use started in the USA almost a decade later in 1974 because of the fear of aplastic anemia. However, once its safety was confirmed, it became the most prescribed AED in the 1980s in Europe and still remains first choice drug for focal onset epilepsy worldwide.

Next in the line was valproate. Valproate was synthesized not as an AED but rather as an organic solvent in 1881 by a chemist Beverly Burton, in the USA; and its anticonvulsant properties were unknown then. Pierre Eymard, who worked at Firma Berthier Laboratories in Grenoble, accidentally discovered anticonvulsant properties of valproate almost 80 years later.[5] Because valproic acid was a liquid, it was used as a lipophilic vehicle to dissolve water-insoluble compounds during preclinical drug testing. Eymard had synthesized a number of khellin derivatives in the laboratory as part of his thesis. In order to evaluate the pharmacological activities of the khellin derivatives as tranquilizing agents in the rat, Carraz (one of the colleagues of Eymard) proposed to test the most active derivatives in the pentylenetetrazole (PTZ) seizure test. Apparently, all agents were found to have anticonvulsant properties. Meunier (another colleague of Eymard) dissolved a coumarin derivative in valproate to find an anticonvulsant effect in the PTZ test in rabbits. By doing this, the researchers found that it was the vehicle, valproate, which exerted an anticonvulsant effect rather than the primary drug tested.[6] This unexpected finding was first presented at a meeting of the French Society of Therapeutics and Pharmacodynamics on December 19, 1962, and published by Meunier, Carraz and Eymard in the French journal Thérapie in 1963.[7] It was marketed in France in 1967 and other European countries in 1970 as an AED. However, its marketing was delayed in the USA until 1978 owing to regulatory monitoring by FDA about the use of new drugs (following the thalidomide disaster). A drug named trimethadione, which was an oxazolidinedione compound, was originally identified as a specific treatment for absence epilepsy by Lennox in 1945.[8] However, owing to its toxic and teratogenic effects, a research was initiated by Parke and Davis which led to the development of ethosuximide. Zimmerman and Burgemeister in 1958 were the first to report its effect in 109 cases of petit mal epilepsy after which it was marketed in 1958 for absence epilepsy.[7]

The major landmark in the history of epilepsy was the discovery of benzodiazepines. Credit for the same goes to Leo Sternbach, a polish Jewish chemist. While working for Hoffmann-La Roche in Nutley, New Jersey, he discovered Valium (diazepam) in 1963.[9] This popular sedative became the most prescribed drug in the United States after its approval in 1963. Known as "mother's little helper", or simply as V, nearly 2.3 billion Valium pills were sold in 1978.[10] This earned tremendous profits for Roche making it a pharmaceutical giant. However, its antiepileptic properties were not harnessed until 1965 when Gastaut used diazepam for successfully treating a patient of status epilepticus after which it became a drug of choice for status epilepticus.[11]

THE ERA OF NEWER AEDS

After this came the era of newer AEDs. National Institute of Neurological Disorders and Stroke (NINDS) in the United States established the Anticonvulsant Drug Development Program in the year 1975. More than 28,000 chemicals were screened since then for anticonvulsant efficacy. Zonisamide was discovered by Uno et al. in 1972 in Japan during exploratory research on psychiatric drugs, where it was subsequently identified as having anticonvulsant activity during screening.[12] Topiramate was discovered in 1979 by Bruce E Maryanoff and Joseph F Gardocki during their research work at McNeil Pharmaceuticals. Discovered accidently in the search for a sugar sulfamate in an antidiabetic project, topiramate was first introduced into clinical practice in 1995 and received United States Food and Drug Administration approval in 1996.[13]

Recently in 2012, topiramate got FDA approval for weight loss along with phentermine. Levetiracetam, which is ethyl analog of piracetam, was synthesized in 1974 by UCB Pharma as a second generation nootropic drug. However, levetiracetam did not show any significant nootropic activity. Rather it showed protection against seizure activity in the genetically sound-sensitive mouse model, suggesting potential antiepileptic properties in humans.[14] However, levetiracetam was the drug which challenged conventional wisdom in AED discovery owing to its unique and unconventional mechanism of action. This prompted a change in the screening models employed both by the NIH and the pharmaceutical industry. All traditional AEDs were tested against two conventional screening models, viz., maximal electroshock seizure test and the pentylenetetrazol test. However, levetiracetam did not show any anticonvulsant properties in these two models. Rather, it effectively controlled seizures in rodents who had chronic epilepsies.[14]

Lamotrigine was originally synthesized by scientists at Wellcome Laboratories. In the mid-1960s, folate was considered a proconvulsant agent and the suggestion that many AEDs were folic acid antagonists, a drug discovery program was initiated keeping in reference pyrimethamine, a folic acid antagonist, previously developed for the treatment of malaria. Among the series of compounds developed, lamotrigine had the most anticonvulsant activity in animal models, although it was a weak inhibitor of dihydrofolate reductase.[15] After extensive clinical trials, it was approved for use in epilepsy in 1990 in Ireland. In 1994, the FDA approved lamotrigine for adjunctive use in epilepsy in the US. Lacosamide was discovered by Dr Harold Kohn, Dr Shridhar Andurkar and colleagues at the University of Houston in 1996. They hypothesized that modified amino acids may be therapeutically useful in the treatment of epilepsy. A few hundred such molecules were synthesized over several years and these were tested in rats. N-benzyl-2-acetamido-3-methoxypropionamide was found to be highly efficacious, which was later renamed lacosamide after being licensed by Schwarz Pharma.[16]

Traditionally antiepileptic medication targeted sodium channels, calcium channels, and inhibitory GABA pathways. Excitatory neurotransmitters like glutamate were considered new targets for development for new AEDs. This led to the formulation of AMPA (glutamate receptor) antagonist perampanel, which is the latest AED approved for the treatment of epilepsy in the year 2016. The development of earlier AMPA receptor antagonists was hindered by poor blood-brain barrier permeability, structure-related toxicity, and short half-lives. Perampanel was discovered as a result of high-throughput screening campaigns, which addressed these shortcomings.[17]

REFERENCES

1. Pearce J. Bromide, the first effective antiepileptic agent. J Neurol Neurosurg Psychiatry. 2002;72(3):412.
2. Friedlander W. The rise and fall of bromide therapy in epilepsy. Arch Neurol. 2000;57(12):1782.
3. Hauptmann A. Luminal bei Epilepsie. Munch Med Wochenshr. 1912;59:1907-9.
4. Brodie M. Antiepileptic drug therapy the story so far. Seizure. 2010;19(10):650-5.
5. Löscher W. The discovery of valproate. Valproate. 1999. pp. 1-3.
6. Shorvon S. Drug treatment of epilepsy in the century of the ILAE: The second 50 years, 1959-2009. Epilepsia. 2009;50:93-130.
7. Meunier H, Carraz G, Neunier Y, et al. Pharmacodynamic properties of N-dipropylacetic acid. Therapie. 1963;18:435-8.
8. Rosenblum J. Trimethadione (Tridione) Nephrosis. Arch Pediatr Adolesc Med. 1959;97(6):790.
9. Wick J. The History of Benzodiazepines. Consult Pharma. 2013;28(9):538-48.
10. Calcaterra N, Barrow J. Classics in Chemical Neuroscience: Diazepam (Valium). ACS Chem Neurosci. 2014;5(4):253-60.
11. Gastaut H, Naquet R, Poiré R, et al. Treatment of Status Epilepticus with Diazepam (Valium). Epilepsia. 1965;6(2):167-82.
12. Uno H, Kurokawa M, Masuda Y, et al. Studies on 3-substituted 1,2-benzisoxazole derivatives. 6. Syntheses of 3-(sulfamoylmethyl)-1,2-benzisoxazole derivatives and their anticonvulsant activities. J Med Chem. 1979;22(2):180-3.
13. Shank R, Gardocki J, Streeter A, et al. An overview of the preclinical aspects of topiramate: pharmacology, pharmacokinetics, and mechanism of action. Epilepsia. 2000;41(s1):3-9.
14. Klitgaard H, Verdru P. Levetiracetam: the first SV2A ligand for the treatment of epilepsy. Expert Opin Drug Discov. 2007;2(11):1537-45.
15. Weisler R, Calabrese J, Bowden C, et al. Discovery and development of lamotrigine for bipolar disorder: A story of serendipity, clinical observations, risk taking, and persistence. J Affect Disord. 2008;108(1-2):1-9.
16. Rogawski M, Tofighy A, White H, et al. Current understanding of the mechanism of action of the antiepileptic drug lacosamide. Epilepsy Res. 2015;110:189-205.
17. Hanada T. The discovery and development of perampanel for the treatment of epilepsy. Expert Opin Drug Discov. 2014;9(4):449-58.

2
CHAPTER

Pharmacology of Antiepileptic Drugs

Atma Ram Bansal, Dinesh Nayak

INTRODUCTION

Pharmacological properties of any drug have two properties—pharmacokinetics and pharmacodynamics.

Pharmacokinetic includes drug absorption, distribution, metabolism and excretion, i.e. what body does to the drug while pharmacodynamics refers to the pharmacological effects of the drug including therapeutic and adverse effects, i.e. what drug does to the body. In this chapter, we have discussed the pharmacological properties of antiepileptic drugs (AEDs). Each drug is discussed in detail in the chapter. From the availability point of view, AEDs can be classified in three groups—older (first-generation) AEDs, newer (second-generation) AEDs and third-generation AEDs. Table 1 describes this classification in detail. AEDs can also be classified based upon mechanism of action (Table 2).

TABLE 1: Three generations of antiepileptic drugs (AEDs) over the century.

First-generation AEDs (1857–1975)	Second-generation AEDs (1993–2007)	Third-generation AEDs (2008–2016)
• Bromides	• Felbamate	• Lacosamide
• Phenobarbitone	• Gabapentin	• Rufinamide
• Phenytoin	• Lamotrigine	• Vigabatrin
• Primidone	• Topiramate	• Eslicarbazepine
• Ethosuximide	• Tiagabine	• Retigabine (ezogabine)
• Diazepam	• Levetiracetam	• Perampanel
• Carbamazepine	• Oxcarbazepine	• Brivaracetam
• Sodium valproate	• Zonisamide	• Stiripentol
• Clonazepam	• Pregabalin	
	• Clobazam	

TABLE 2: Mechanism of action of various antiepileptic drugs.

Sodium channel actions	
Blockade by stabilizing fast inactivated state	Phenytoin, carbamazepine, lamotrigine, oxcarbazepine, rufinamide, eslicarbazepine
Blockade by stabilizing slow inactivated state	Lacosamide
Calcium channel actions	
Blockade of high voltage-activated channel (P/Q type)	Gabapentin, pregabalin
Blockade of low voltage-activated channel (T type)	Ethosuximide
GABA-related actions	
Activation of GABAA receptor	Phenobarbitone, benzodiazepines
Blockade of GABA transporter (GAT1a selective)	Tiagabine
Inhibition of GABA transaminase	Vigabatrin
SV2A (synaptic vesicle) actions	
Modulation of SV2A	Levetiracetam, brivaracetam
Multiple actions	
Various actions on multiple targets	Valproic acid, felbamate, topiramate, zonisamide
Potassium channel activity	
Opens Kv7 potassium channels	Retigabine/ezogabine
Glutamate blockade via NMDA receptor	
Blockade of the postsynaptic excitatory AMPA receptor	Felbamate
Glutamate blockade via AMPA receptor	
Blockade of the postsynaptic excitatory AMPA receptor	Perampanel

ANTIEPILEPTIC DRUGS

Phenobarbitone

Phenobarbitone is the first effective and the least expensive AED currently used in neurological practice. It was first discovered as hypnotic agent in 1912.[1] Phenobarbitone exerts its antiepileptic action by facilitating gamma-aminobutyric acid (GABA) receptor-mediated inhibition. It extends the mean open duration of the GABAA receptor (GABAAR), thereby increasing Cl^- flux. Increased intracellular chloride results in hyperpolarization of the postsynaptic neuronal membrane, which helps in interrupting the spread of epileptic activity.[2] It has very good bioavailability (80–100%) with oral or intramuscular (IM) use of in adults.[3] Phenobarbitone is primarily having hepatic metabolism and nearly 25% is excreted via kidney as unchanged drug, which is sensitive to urine pH.[4] Phenobarbitone is an enzyme inducer and can interact with other AEDs as well as antitubercular drugs and oral anticoagulation. Plasma protein binding is 40–60%. Among AEDs, it is having highest T½ of 65–110 hours.[5] With intravenous use, it is distributed very quickly to highly vascular organs, except the brain, which takes about 6-12 minutes, penetration in brain is much faster during status epilepticus. Serum phenobarbital concentrations should be checked 3–4 weeks after the initial dose, with a goal therapeutic level of 10–40 μg/mL (43–172 μmol/L). Side effects of phenobarbitone include hyperactivity, behavioral problems, sedation, and even dementia especially in elderly.[6] Some of these effects may be related to dose as well.

Phenytoin

Phenytoin (diphenylhydantoin) was introduced in 1938.[7] It blocks sodium channels thus affecting the propagation of the action potential and post-tetanic potentiation, which affect onset and spread of seizures.[8] It also has an inhibiting effect on calcium-calmodulin protein phosphorylation. It is not absorbed low pH of the gastric juices but absorbed in the small intestines with a higher pH. Phenytoin also has very good bioavailability after oral intake (95–100%) and T½ is 7–42 hours (mean—22 hours) and hence can be taken once a day, and peak level after oral administration is reached in approximately 4–12 hours. It is highly plasma protein bound (90–95%). It is mainly having renal excretion but not affected by hemodialysis due to high protein binding. It is metabolized in liver by P450 enzymes. It is a strong enzyme inducer as well. It results in significant drug interaction with other drugs. Due to nonlinear pharmacokinetics, any small change in doses can significantly affect drug level resulting in a very narrow therapeutic index.[9,10] There can be significant difference in various brands and generic preparations in phenytoin content, which can seizure control or result in toxicity when patients are switched from one preparation to another one.[11]

Side effects of phenytoin include allergic reaction, nausea and vomiting, blood dyscrasias, vitamin and hormonal dysfunction, and bone marrow hypoplasia. Phenytoin is still one of the most common drugs used by primary care physician in view of a very old and effective drug with once daily dosing and availability of parenteral preparation.

For intravenous use, fosphenytoin sodium, a phosphate ester prodrug of phenytoin, is a better choice, as it is rapidly absorbed by the IM and intravenous (IV) route.[12] It has fewer side effects (including cardiovascular depression and hypotension) than phenytoin. Fosphenytoin is not excreted in the urine.

Sodium Valproate

Sodium valproate (VPA) is one of the most commonly used first generation AEDs with very broad spectrum coverage. It is weak acid and insoluble in water, but its sodium salt is freely water soluble. VPA is having excellent bioavailability, close to 100% with rapid and near total absorption.

Mechanism of Action

Sodium VPA acts as AED by various mechanisms.[13] VPA blocks voltage-dependent sodium channels causing suppression of high frequency, repetitive neuronal firing. It also enhances GABA function, but this effect is observed only at high concentrations. It may increase the synthesis of GABA by stimulating glutamate decarboxylase (GAD). Its weak action on T-type calcium currents is useful in absence of epilepsy. Valproic acid is extensively bound to plasma proteins (>90%). It is having nonlinear kinetics due to short T½ (12–20 hours) and concentration-dependent protein binding.[14] It competes with itself for protein binding, which leads to a nonlinear increase in total concentration and relatively lower concentration at higher doses.[15] Valproic acid is also an inhibitor of cytochrome P4502C19.[16] It is extensively metabolized in the liver (96%) and about 4% is excreted unchanged in urine. It is a potent enzyme inhibitor and results in increased concentration of other drugs.

Common side effects of VPA include weight gain, gastrointestinal (GI) disturbance, hair loss and tremor. Hormonal disturbance includes menstrual irregularity, polycystic ovarian disease (PCOD) and insulin resistance.[17] Other uncommon but significant side effects include hepatotoxicity, acute pancreatitis and thrombocytopenia, and other coagulation disturbances.[18]

Carbamazepine

Carbamazepine (CBZ) is a very effective drug in focal seizures. It was initially used for trigeminal neuralgia and incidentally detected to have antiepileptic action. It acts on voltage-dependent sodium channels resulting in inhibition of the generation of rapid action potentials and prevention of post-tetanic potentiation. Being a crystalline substance, it is insoluble in water and hence only oral preparations are available. Its bioavailability is about 80%, T½ is 6–12 hours, and plasma protein binding is 70–85%. It has hepatic metabolism by cytochrome P450 (CYP) 3A4 and is also a very potent and broad-spectrum inducer of the CYP system resulting in significant drug interaction.

Because CBZ induces its own metabolism (autoinduction), it is important to titrate the doses over about 4 weeks.[15] It may be important to check the blood levels at 2–3 months to see for maintenance doses of CBZ. Most important side effects include allergic rash, pruritis and even Stevens–Johnson syndrome. It is advisable to check for HLA-B*1502 allele before starting CBZ especially in Asian population.[19] Other systemic side effects include nausea, vomiting, diarrhea, hyponatremia and fluid retention. Drug overdose may result in dizziness, diplopia and ataxia. Rare idiosyncratic adverse effects include bone marrow depression.

Benzodiazepines

These were initially developed as anxiolytic agents in the 1950s. There are four drugs used in epilepsy. Lorazepam and diazepam are mainly used in acute treatment of seizures, while clonazepam and diazepam are used as long-term AEDs. The GABAAR is a major target of benzodiazepines. They act by binding between the alpha and gamma subunits of the GABA receptor, potentiating GABA-mediated inhibition of neurotransmission.[20] The 1,5-benzodiazepines are less lipophilic and acidic than the 1,4-benzodiazepines, changing their distribution characteristics and potentially resulting in less sedation and a slower development of tolerance.

Clobazam

It is available only in oral formulations because of water-insoluble compound. Clobazam displays linear and dose-independent pharmacokinetics.[21] Clobazam is rapidly and almost completely absorbed and reaches its peak within 0.5–4 hours. Administration with food does not affect the rate or extent of absorption.[22] Clobazam is 80–90% protein bound. The half-life of the clobazam is 18 hours. Its main active metabolite, N-desmethylclobazam, attains maximal plasma concentration after 24–72 hours.[23] Clobazam has no enzyme inducing or inhibiting property and so has no major drug interaction.[21]

There is an apprehension about tolerance of antiseizure action of benzodiazepines including clobazam, but recent studies have clearly documented significant long-term retention and efficacy of clobazam without changes in doses.[24]

In patients greater than 2 years of age, clobazam may be started at 5 mg/day in one dose, typically given at bedtime. The dose may be increased in intervals no shorter than every 7 days to a maximum of 40 mg/day in a divided schedule (maximum 20 mg/day for weight ≤30 kg). Side effects of clobazam include sedation, constipation, lethargy, drooling, aggression and irritability, and weight gain.[25,26]

Clonazepam

It is effective mainly in myoclonic seizures and subcortical myoclonus. It acts on GABA receptor. In addition, there is some action on sodium channels. It is rapidly and almost completely (more than 90%) absorbed after oral administration. It is highly metabolized in liver and only less than 2% unchanged clonazepam is excreted in the urine.

Plasma protein binding is approximately 86%. It is highly lipid soluble and can cross the blood–brain barrier rapidly. Plasma levels and antiepileptic effects are not correlated. Clonazepam has dose-independent pharmacokinetics without any autoinduction or interaction with other drugs. Major side effect of clonazepam is sedation, which is more common in adults than children. Other side effects include hyperactivity, respiratory depression and hypersalivation.

It is an effective drug for management of status epilepticus,[27] though IV form is not available in India. It is important to taper the benzodiazepines including clonazepam very slowly as withdrawal may increase the risk of exacerbation of seizures or even status epilepticus. Other withdrawal symptoms may include insomnia, anxiety, psychosis and tremor.

Midazolam

Its main use is in status epilepticus, as it has a rapid onset and short duration of action. It is used as bolus as well as continuous IV infusion. Its salt is water soluble. It is rapidly eliminated from the body within 1–3 hours.[28] Intranasal midazolam is very effective for prehospital treatment of status epilepticus and it can be used as a rescue medicine in patients with severe epilepsy.[29] It is rapidly absorbed as mucosal surface of nasopharynx is large and well vascularized. High first-pass metabolism is also avoided by nasal route.[30]

Lorazepam

It is drug of choice as first-line antiepileptic for status epilepticus due to rapid onset and sustained antiepileptic action.[31] It is rapidly and readily absorbed and reaches its peak within 2 hours after oral administration.

NEWER ANTIEPILEPTIC DRUGS

Levetiracetam

A piracetam derivative (S)-α-ethyl-2-oxo-1-pyrrolidineacetamide was approved by the Food and Drug Administration in the year 1999.[32] Its mechanism of action is different from other AEDs, as it does not act on GABA, sodium, or calcium channels but binds to the synaptic vesicle protein SV2A and modulates synaptic transmission through alteration of vesicle fusion.[33] SV2A is important for the availability of calcium-dependent neurotransmitter vesicles ready to release their content.[34]

It is neither metabolized by cytochrome system nor it induces or inhibits this system and hence is having practically no significant drug interaction. It is rapidly and completely absorbed after oral administration though food can delay the abruption. It does not bind to plasma protein and almost two-third is excreted unchanged by kidney.[35] A dose adjustment is recommended for moderate-to-severe renal impairment or severe hepatic impairment with concomitant renal insufficiency. It is equally effective in children.[36] As parenteral formulations are available, it is commonly used in critical care settings and status epilepticus.[37] The most common side effects of levetiracetam include neurobehavioral symptoms like nervousness, irritability, agitation, aggression, emotional lability, depression and mood swings. These symptoms may be severe enough to cause discontinuation of the medications in some patients.[38]

Lamotrigine

Lamotrigine (LTG) is a triazine compound that is chemically unrelated to any of the other AEDs. It was initially developed as antifolate agent. Mechanism of action is by blocking voltage-gated sodium channel, but it also inhibits release of glutamate by selectively influencing neurons that synthesize glutamate and aspartate.[39] Being water and ethanol insoluble, it is available only in oral formulations with a complete absorption. It is metabolized by liver and has a plasma protein binding of about 55%. Drugs like sodium VPA with enzyme inhibition property increase drug level of LTG, while enzyme-inducing drugs like phenytoin decrease its level, however, LTG per se does not induce or inhibit hepatic enzymes. Due to increased clearance during pregnancy (>50%), there is a significant drop in serum level of LTG, which comes back to normal in postpartum period and hence dose adjustments are required during pregnancy and postpartum period.[40,41]

Lamotrigine is effective in almost all types of epilepsies but can exaggerate myoclonus. Most significant side effect is drug allergy, which can even result in Stevens-Johnson syndrome, so a slow titration is advised. In patients with initially allergy, a rechallenge with further slower titration can be done.[42] Other side effects include dizziness, diplopia, ataxia and somnolence. Rare cases (about 40 patients) of aseptic meningitis are reported in patients taking LTG.[43]

Topiramate

It was initially developed as antidiabetic drug but was found to have potent antiepileptic effect. It has multiple mechanisms of action including sodium channels, GABA receptors and glutamate receptors. In addition, it has weak action on carbonic anhydrase. It has a rapid and near total absorption after oral intake with bioavailability close to 100%. Only 15% of topiramate is metabolized in the liver by the P450 microsomal enzyme system and 85% is excreted unchanged in the kidney. Due to delayed excretion in renal diseases, a reduction in usual dose is recommended for moderate-to-severe renal impairment. Due to low plasma protein binding (15%), a supplement dose may be required during hemodialysis.[44] Dose adjustments might not be required in moderate-to-severe hepatic impairments. Topiramate has no significant drug interaction with other drugs but enzyme-inducing drugs can decrease its serum levels.[45]

It is used for all types of seizures and is also a very effective drug for migraine prophylaxis. Side effects include impaired cognition and expressive language, which can result in discontinuation of therapy.[46] Other side effects of topiramate include paresthesias, headache, fatigue, dizziness, depression and mood problems. Decreased sweating with topiramate may lead to heat intolerance and hyperthermia, particularly in children.

Rare but severe adverse effect includes acute myopia and secondary angle glaucoma, resulting in acute onset of decreased visual acuity and/or ocular pain.[47] It usually happens within 1 month of initiating treatment and warrants immediate discontinuation of the drug. Renal stone is another side effect for which a baseline ultrasound may be recommended in high-risk patients.[48] In view of side effect of weight loss, it may be considered as a good choice AED for obese patients.

Zonisamide

It is a sulfonamide derivative that is structurally related to antibiotics. Its primary mechanism of action includes voltage-dependent sodium and T-type calcium channels. Like topiramate, it is also a weak inhibitor of carbonic anhydrase. It has a rapid and complete absorption after oral administration and has a very long T½ of around 60 hours and hence can be taken in once daily doses. It has a linear kinetics and has 40–50% plasma protein binding.[49] It is metabolized by cytochrome 450 and hence its level is affected by enzyme-inducing drugs.[50] Zonisamide does not have significant drug interaction with other drugs. Because of significant renal excretion, it should be given cautiously in patients with renal impairment. Like topiramate, it is effective in all types of epilepsies including myoclonic epilepsy. Side effects of zonisamide include drowsiness, anorexia, behavioral and cognitive disturbance. Some of side effects like decrease sweating, renal stone and weight loss are similar to topiramate.

Lacosamide

It is used for refractory focal epilepsy as well as status epilepticus (especially recurrent focal seizures). It has novel mechanism of action and selectively enhances slow inactivation of voltage-gated sodium channels. It affects sustained firing of epileptic neurons by regulating the long-term availability of these channels.[51] It also has a rapid and complete absorption after oral intake, which is unaffected by food intake. It has very low plasma protein binding (15%) and is metabolized by liver and primarily excreted via kidney. Its level is minimally affected by mild-to-moderate renal impairment, while it should be used cautiously in severe renal and hepatic dysfunction. It has negligible drug interaction with other AEDs and systemic drugs. Lacosamide intravenous solution is typically administered over 30 minutes. Commonly reported side effects include dizziness, headache, nausea and diplopia. It has no significant cardiac side effects including change in heart rate, QTc interval or QRS duration. A small but clinically insignificant increase in mean PR interval at the end of maintenance (1.4–6.6 ms increase), which is similar to other AEDs.[52]

Oxcarbazepine

It is similar to CBZ in structure, mechanism of action, and efficacy. It is the 10-ketoanalogue of CBZ but with better pharmacokinetic profile as there is no autoinduction and fewer drug interactions.[53] Unlike CBZ, it does not produce epoxide metabolite, which is responsible for side effects. CBZ can be abruptly substituted with an oxcarbazepine (OXC) with an OXC:CBZ ratio of 3:2. Side effects include somnolence, dizziness, rash, hyponatremia, weight gain, nausea and alopecia.[54] The incidence of hyponatremia associated with OXC therapy may be higher than that seen with CBZ especially in elderly.[55] OXC level may decrease during pregnancy and increase after delivery and hence a dose adjustment is required to avoid seizure recurrence or drug toxicity.

Eslicarbazepine

Eslicarbazepine is a third-generation drug of dibenz[b,f]azepine family of AEDs, which includes CBZ (first generation) and OXC (second generation). OXC is metabolized to both R- and the S-licarbazepine, eslicarbazepine acetate is rapidly converted, primarily to S-licarbazepine (also known as eslicarbazepine), and is generally undetectable in serum as the parent compound.[56] It has a better pharmacokinetics with a linear pharmacokinetics, very low potential for drug–drug interactions and once daily dosing. Side effect profile is almost similar except that hyponatremia is less.[57]

Ethosuximide

It acts on T-type calcium currents in thalamic neurons and is the drug of choice for absence seizures; however, it is ineffective in focal and generalized tonic-clonic seizures.[58] It is not available in India. It has been used since early 1950s as an AED for the treatment of absence seizures.[59] It is readily absorbed from the GI tract. Enzyme-inducing AEDs can reduce the level of ethosuximide. In refractory absence seizures, it can be used in combination with VPA.[60] There are no major side effects except some degree of GI and sleep disturbance.

Vigabatrin

Vigabatrin is a structural analog of the inhibitory neurotransmitter GABA. It is being used as AED since 1979,[61] but was approved by FDA in 2009 as add-on drug for refractory focal seizures and as monotherapy for infantile spasms. It is rapidly and completely absorbed after oral intake and food does not inhibit absorption. It has no plasma protein binding. Its T½ is 3–5 hours and excreted mainly by kidney. It has no major drug interaction with AEDs except that it can reduce phenytoin level probably by decreasing absorption.[62] It acts by irreversibly inhibiting the degradative enzyme GABA-transaminase and thus increasing central nervous system GABA levels. It is a very effective for infantile spasms[63] and is the treatment of choice in infantile spasms associated with tuberous sclerosis.[64] Vigabatrin may worsen myoclonic and absences and hence should be avoided in primary generalized epilepsies. The most significant side effect is visual field constriction and hence periodic field charting is advised in children more than 9 years of cognitive age.[65] Other side effects include drowsiness, confusion, weight gain, sleep disturbance and excitation.[66]

Gabapentin

Though it has chemical structural similar to GABA but it has no action on GABA receptors. It mainly acts via voltage-sensitive calcium channels and some effect on glutamate. Gabapentin is a safe and well-tolerated drug with unique pharmacokinetic profile and broad-therapeutic index. It has dose-dependent oral absorption at high dosages and has no plasma protein binding with primary elimination by the kidney. It has no significant drug interaction with other AEDs. It is effective for newly diagnosed focal epilepsy; however, there is insufficient evidence to recommend its use in refractory partial epilepsy.[67] Its efficacy is modest especially at lower doses and hence is not being used as an AED very frequently. Side effects include dizziness and drowsiness. It can worsen myoclonic seizures.

Pregabalin

Its pharmacokinetic and pharmacodynamic profile is similar to gabapentin except that it has more rapid absorption and linear pharmacokinetics.[68] Pregabalin is more effective for neuropathic pain. It is well tolerated and can be used as an adjunctive therapy for focal seizures, with or without secondary generalizations.[69]

Perampanel

Perampanel is a selective noncompetitive AMPA (α-amino-3-hydroxy-5-methyl-4-isoxazolepropionic acid) receptor (of glutamate) antagonist.[70] It has a very long T½ and hence can be given in OD doses. It is rapidly and completely absorbed by GI tract, though food can delay absorption. It has linear pharmacokinetics. It has significant plasma protein binding to the range of 90–95% and only remaining drug exerts pharmacological effect. It is extensively metabolized in liver and hence enzyme-inducing drugs can cause decrease in drug level. It can have significant side effects like psychiatric and behavioral adverse reactions like irritability, anger, and aggression. Other side effects include dullness, gait disturbance, weight gain, dysarthria and euphoric mood.[71] It was approved by FDA for use as an adjuvant treatment in focal seizures in 2012 and in generalized tonic-clonic seizures in 2015. The starting dose is 2 mg/day and then target dose is 8–12 mg/day.

Retigabine

It is a novel drug that opens voltage-sensitive potassium channels that decrease neuronal excitability. However, recently, some action on GABA receptors has also been reported.[72] It has been approved by FDA in 2011 for the adjunctive treatment of focal seizures. It can exert inhibitory effects on potassium channels in the urogenital tract, which can lead to urinary retention, usually within 6 months of treatment.[73] Other side effects include discoloration of skin, conjunctiva and sclera, ataxia, dizziness, fatigue and nausea.[74,75]

Rufinamide

Rufinamide, a triazole derivative, acts on sodium channels by reducing the recovery capacity after inactivation and limiting action potential firing.[76] It is used as adjunctive therapy in with Lennox-Gastaut syndrome in patients aged more than or equal to 4 years.[77] It has fewer drug-drug interactions. Side effects include dizziness, fatigue, lethargy and headache.[78]

Stiripentol

It acts on GABA receptors and is effective for myoclonic seizures. It is especially used in severe myoclonic epilepsy of infancy—Dravet syndrome.[79] It is not yet approved by FDA.

Tiagabine

It is a newer AED and acts by inhibiting presynaptic and glial uptake of GABA. It is reported to be effective in patients with drug-resistant focal epilepsy. Adverse effects include dizziness, nervousness and tremor.[80]

Brivaracetam

Brivaracetam is a more potent analog of levetiracetam with a significantly higher affinity for SVA2 protein (30 times).[81] It was approved by FDA in 2016 and was launched in India in 2017.[82] Other pharmacological properties like bioavailability, plasma protein binding, renal excretion, and half life are similar to levetiracetam. Dose of brivaracetam is $1/10^{th}$ to $1/15^{th}$ of levetiracetam and can be switched overnight. It is given in doses of 50–150 mg/day. Its behavioral side effects are claimed to be lesser than levetiracetam.

PHARMACOLOGICAL PROPERTIES OF ANTIEPILEPTIC DRUGS

Various pharmacological properties of AEDs are summarized in Table 3.

PHARMACOKINETIC PROPERTIES OF ANTIEPILEPTIC DRUGS

Various pharmacokinetic properties of AEDs are described in Table 4.

SIDE EFFECTS OF ANTIEPILEPTIC DRUGS

Side effects of AEDs are summarized in Table 5.

CONCLUSION

With the advancement in the discovery of newer antiepileptic drugs, its important to have an updated knowledge of pharmacology of these drugs. This helps in understanding drug doses, drug interaction and side effects. Various tables given above in the chapter are of utmost importance as a ready reference. The other chapters in the book will cover individual drug and its indication along with the drug of choice in various type of epilepsy. The pharmacological properties will be beneficial in understanding combination therapy which is covered in a separate chapter.

TABLE 3: Dosage, therapeutic drug levels and enzyme induction properties of antiepileptic drugs (AEDs).

AEDs	Dosage (mg/kg/day)	Half life (hours)	Dosage	Daily maintenance dose (mg/day)	Daily maximum dose (mg/day)	Enzyme induction
Phenobarbitone	3–8	60–110	OD	60–90	180	Yes
Phenytoin	5–8	20–40	OD	300	500	Yes
Carbamazepine	10–30	12–17	BD	600–800	1,600	Yes
Valproate	20–60	8–17	BD	400–800	1,600	Inhibition
Oxcarbazepine	20–45	10–15	BD	600–900	2,400	Yes
Lamotrigine	5–15	15–60	BD	200	500	No
Topiramate	3–9	12–30	BD	200	400	Yes (weak)
Zonisamide	5–8	50–70	OD	200	400	No
Levetiracetam	20–80	6–8	BD	1,000	3,000	No
Lacosamide	4–8	12–16	BD	200	400	No
Eslicarbazepine	8–12	20–24	OD	400	800	Yes (weak)
Clobazam	0.5–1	20–40	OD	10	40	No
Rufinamide	20–60	6–10	BD	800	1,200	Yes
Perampanel	–	105	OD	4–8	12	No
Brivaracetam	2	8	BD	100	200	No

TABLE 4: Pharmacokinetic properties of antiepileptic drugs (AEDs).

AEDs	Absorption	Elimination route	Protein binding	Drug interaction
Phenobarbitone	100%	75% hepatic	50%	Yes
Phenytoin	95%	100% hepatic	70–95%	Yes
Carbamazepine	80%	100% hepatic	75–80%	Yes
Valproate	100%	90% hepatic	85–95%	Yes
Oxcarbazepine	100%	100% hepatic	40%	Yes
Lamotrigine	98%	100% hepatic	55%	Yes
Topiramate	>80%	30–55% renal	15%	Yes
Zonisamide	80–100%	50–70% hepatic	40–60%	No
Levetiracetam	100%	66% renal	<10%	No
Lacosamide	100%	95% renal	<15%	No
Eslicarbazepine	>90%	90% renal	<40%	Yes
Clobazam	87–100%	94% renal	80–90%	No
Rufinamide	85%	85% renal	34%	Yes
Perampanel	100%	70% hepatic	95%	Yes
Brivaracetam	100%	95% renal	20%	No

TABLE 5: Common adverse effects of antiepileptic drugs (AEDs).

AEDs	Adverse effects
Phenobarbitone	Sedation, depression and paradoxical hyperactivity
Phenytoin	Ataxia, hirsutism, gingival hyperplasia, nystagmus, lupus-like reaction, osteomalacia and folate deficiency
Carbamazepine	Rash, diplopia, Stevens–Johnson syndrome, hyponatremia, leukopenia and ataxia
Valproate	Hepatotoxicity, hyperammonemia, thrombocytopenia, weight gain and hair fall
Oxcarbazepine	Hyponatremia, dizziness, ataxia and rash
Lamotrigine	Stevens–Johnson syndrome, hypersensitivity and rash
Topiramate	Renal calculi, word finding difficulty, metabolic acidosis, hypohidrosis, paresthesias, weight loss, acute glaucoma and depression
Zonisamide	Renal calculi, weight loss, rash, Stevens–Johnson syndrome and fatigue
Levetiracetam	Irritability, behavioral issues and psychosis
Lacosamide	Dizziness and nausea
Eslicarbazepine	Fatigue, nausea, dizziness and ataxia
Clobazam	Sedation and salivation
Rufinamide	Loss of appetite, vomiting and fatigue
Perampanel	Irritability, mood swings, homicidal ideations and dizziness
Brivaracetam	Irritability and behavioral changes

REFERENCES

1. López-Muñoz F, Ucha-Udabe R, Alamo C. The history of barbiturates a century after their clinical introduction. Neuropsychiatr Dis Treat. 2005;1(4):329-43.
2. Anderson GD. Phenobarbital and other barbiturates: chemistry, biotransformation, and pharmacokinetics. In: Levy RH, Mattson RH, Meldrum BS, Perucca E (Eds). Antiepileptic Drugs, 5th edition. Philadelphia: Lippincott Williams & Wilkins; 2002. pp. 496-503.
3. Rogawski MA. Diverse mechanisms of antiepileptic drugs in the development pipeline. Epilepsy Res. 2006;69(3):273-94.
4. Michelucchi R, Pasini E, Tassinari CA. Phenobarbital, primidone and other barbiturates. In: Shorvon S, Perucca E, Engel Jr (Eds). The treatment of epilepsy, 3rd edition. USA: Wiley-Blackwell; 2009. pp. 585-604.
5. Bourgeois BF. Important pharmacokinetic properties of antiepileptic drugs. Epilepsia. 1995;36 Suppl 5:S1-7.
6. Iivanainen M, Savolainen H. Side effects of phenobarbital and phenytoin during long-term treatment of epilepsy. Acta Neurol Scand Suppl. 1983;97:49-67.
7. Shorvon SD. Drug treatment of epilepsy in the century of the ILAE: The first 50 years, 1909–1958. Epilepsia. 2009;50(S3):69-92.
8. Yaari Y, Selzer ME, Pincus JH. Phenytoin: mechanisms of its anticonvulsant action. Ann Neurol. 1986;20(2):171-84.
9. Ludden TM. Nonlinear pharmacokinetics: clinical Implications. Clin Pharmacokinet. 1991;20(6):429-46.
10. Perucca E, Dulac O, Shorvon S, et al. Harnessing the clinical potential of anti-epileptic drug therapy: dosage optimisation. CNS Drugs. 2001;15(8):609-21.
11. Soryal I, Richens A. Bioavailability and dissolution of proprietary and generic formulations of phenytoin. J Neurol Neurosurg Psychiatry. 1992;55(8):688-91.
12. Browne TR, Kugler AR, Eldon MA. Pharmacology and pharmacokinetics of fosphenytoin. Neurology. 1996;46(6 Suppl 1):S3-7.
13. Löscher W. Basic pharmacology of valproate: a review after 35 years of clinical use for the treatment of epilepsy. CNS Drugs. 2002;16(10):669-94.
14. Zaccara G, Messori A, Moroni F. Clinical pharmacokinetics of valproic acid. Clin Pharmacokinet. 1988;15(6):367-89.
15. Bourgeois BF. Pharmacokinetic properties of current antiepileptic drugs. Neurology 2000;55(11 Suppl 3):S11-6.
16. Beyenburg S, Bauer J, Reuber M. New drugs for the treatment of epilepsy: a practical approach. Postgrad Med J. 2004;80(948):581-7.
17. Abaci A, Saygi M, Yis U, et al. Metabolic alterations during valproic acid treatment: a prospective study. Pediatr Neurol. 2009;41(6):435-9.
18. Nasreddine W, Beydoun A. Valproate-induced thrombocytopenia: a prospective monotherapy study. Epilepsia. 2008;49(3):438-45.
19. Ferrell PB Jr, McLeod HL. Carbamazepine, HLA-B*1502 and risk of Stevens-Johnson syndrome and toxic epidermal necrolysis: US FDA recommendations. Pharmacogenomics. 2008;9(10):1543-6.
20. Treiman DM. GABAergic mechanisms in epilepsy. Epilepsia. 2001;42(Suppl 3):8-12.
21. Rupp W, Badian M, Christ O, et al. Pharmacokinetics of single and multiple doses of clobazam in humans. Br J Clin Pharmacol. 1979;7(Suppl 1):51-7.
22. Tedeschi G, Riva R. Baruzzi A. Clobazam plasma concentrations: pharmacokinetic study in healthy volunteers and data in epileptic patients. Br J Clin Pharmac. 1981;11(6):619-22.
23. Hanks GW. Clobazam Pharmacological and therapeutic profile. Br J Clin Pharmacol. 1979;7(Suppl 1):151S-155S.
24. Conry JA, Ng YT, Kernitsky L, et al. OV-1004 Study Investigators Stable dosages of clobazam for Lennox-Gastaut syndrome are associated with sustained drop-seizure and total-seizure improvements over 3 years. Epilepsia. 2014;55(4): 558-67.
25. Kalra V, Seth R, Mishra D, et al. Clobazam in refractory childhood epilepsy. Indian J Pedatr. 2010;77(3):263-6.

26. Faulkner MA. Comprehensive overview: efficacy, tolerability, and cost-effectiveness of clobazam in Lennox-Gastaut syndrome. Ther Clin Risk Manag. 2015;8:905-14.
27. Alvarez V, Lee JW, Drislane FW, et al. Practice variability and efficacy of clonazepam, lorazepam, and midazolam in status epilepticus: A multicenter comparison. Epilepsia. 2015;56(8):1275-85.
28. Smith MT, Eadie MJ, Brophy TO. The pharmacokinetics of midazolam in man. Eur J Clin Pharmacol. 1981;19(4):271-8.
29. Scheepers M, Scheepers B, Clarke M, et al. Is intranasal midazolam an effective rescue medication in adolescents and adults with severe epilepsy? Seizure. 2000;9(6):417-21.
30. Knoester PD, Jonker DM, Van Der Hoeven RT, et al. Pharmacokinetics and pharmacodynamics of midazolam administered as a concentrated intranasal spray. A study in healthy volunteers. Br J Clin Pharmacol. 2002;53(5):501-7.
31. Walker M. Status epilepticus: an evidence based guide. BMJ. 2005;331(7518):673-7.
32. Hovinga CA. Levetiracetam: a novel antiepileptic drug. Pharmacotherapy. 2001;21(11):1375-88.
33. Custer KL, Austin NS, Sullivan JM, et al. Synaptic vesicle protein 2 enhances release probability at quiescent synapses. J Neurosci. 2006;26(4):1303-13.
34. Xu T, Bajjalieh SM. SV2 modulates the size of the readily releasable pool of secretory vesicles. Nat Cell Biol. 2001;3(8):691-8.
35. Walker MC, Patsalos PN. Clinical pharmacokinetics of new antiepileptic drugs. Pharmacol Ther. 1995;67(3):351-84.
36. Weijenberg A, Brouwer OF, Callenbach PM. Levetiracetam monotherapy in children with epilepsy: A systematic review. CNS Drugs. 2015;29(5):371-82.
37. DeWolfe JL, Szaflarski JP. Levetiracetam use in the critical care setting. Front Neurol. 2013;4:121.
38. Cramer JA, De Rue K, Devinsky O, et al. A systematic review of the behavioral effects of levetiracetam in adults with epilepsy, cognitive disorders, or an anxiety disorder during clinical trials. Epilepsy Behav. 2003;4:124-32.
39. Lee CY, Fu WM, Chen CC, et al. Lamotrigine inhibits postsynaptic AMPA receptor and glutamate release in the dentate gyrus. Epilepsia. 2008;49(5):888-97.
40. Tran TA, Leppik IE, Blesi K, et al. Lamotrigine clearance during pregnancy. Neurology. 2002;59:251-5.
41. Pennell PB, Peng L, Newport DJ, et al. Lamotrigine in pregnancy: Clearance, therapeutic drug monitoring, and seizure frequency. Neurology. 2008;70(22 Pt 2):2130-6.
42. P-Codrea Tigaran S, Sidenius P, Dam M. Lamotrigine-induced rash—worth a rechallenge. Acta Neurol Scand. 2005;111:191-4.
43. Simms KM, Kortepeter C, Avigan M. Lamotrigine and aseptic meningitis. Neurology. 2012;78:921-7.
44. Manitpisitkul P, Shalayda K, Wang SS, et al. Pharmacokinetics of topiramate in patients with renal impairment, end-stage renal disease undergoing hemodialysis, or hepatic impairment. Epilepsy Res. 2014;108(5):891-901.
45. Bialer M, Doose D, Murthy B, et al. Pharmacokinetic interactions of topiramate. Clin Pharmacokinet. 2004;43:763-80.
46. Cirulli ET, Urban TJ, Marino SE, et al. Genetic and environmental correlates of topiramate-induced cognitive impairment. Epilepsia. 2012;53(1):e5-8.
47. Etminan M, Maberley D, Mikelberg FS. Use of topiramate and risk of glaucoma: a case-control study. Am J Ophthalmol. 2012;153(5):827-30.
48. Mahmoud AA, Rizk T, El-Bakri NK, et al. Incidence of kidney stones with topiramate treatment in pediatric patients. Epilepsia. 2011;52(10):1890-3.
49. Brodie MJ, Ben-Menachem E, Chouette I, et al. Zonisamide: its pharmacology, efficacy and safety in clinical trials. Acta Neurol Scand Suppl. 2012;(194):19-28.
50. Sills G, Brodie M. Pharmacokinetics and drug interactions with zonisamide. Epilepsia. 2007;48:435-41.

51. Errington AC, Stöhr T, Heers C, et al. The investigational anticonvulsant lacosamide selectively enhances slow inactivation of voltage-gated sodium channels. Mol Pharmacol. 2008;73:157-69.
52. Beydoun A, D'Souza J, Hebert D, et al. Lacosamide: pharmacology, mechanisms of action and pooled efficacy and safety data in partial-onset seizures. Expert Rev Neurother. 2009;9:33-42.
53. Grant SM, Faulds D. Oxcarbazepine. A review of its pharmacology and therapeutic potential in epilepsy, trigeminal neuralgia and affective disorders. Drugs. 1992;43:873-88.
54. Buggy Y, Layton D, Fogg C, et al. Safety profile of oxcarbazepine: results from a prescription-event monitoring study. Epilepsia. 2010;51(5):818.
55. Dong X, Leppik IE, White J, et al. Hyponatremia from oxcarbazepine and carbamazepine. Neurology. 2005;65(12):1976-8.
56. Ben-Menachem E. Eslicarbazepine acetate: a well-kept secret? Epilepsy Curr. 2010;10(1):7-8.
57. Gil-Nagel A, Elger C, Ben-Menachem E, et al. Efficacy and safety of eslicarbazepine acetate as add-on treatment in patients with focal-onset seizures: integrated analysis of pooled data from double-blind phase III clinical studies. Epilepsia. 2013;54(1):98-107.
58. Glauser TA, Cnaan A, Shinnar S, et al. Ethosuximide, valproic acid, and lamotrigine in childhood absence epilepsy. N Engl J Med. 2010;362(9):790-9.
59. Giaccone M, Bartoli A, Gatti G, et al. Effect of enzyme inducing anticonvulsants on ethosuximide pharmacokinetics in epileptic patients. Br J Clin Pharmacol. 1996;41(6):575-9.
60. Rowan AJ, Meijer JWA, de Beer-Pawlikowski N, et al. Valproate–ethosuximide combination therapy for refractory absence seizures. Arch Neurol. 1983;40(13): 797-802.
61. French JA. Vigabatrin. Epilepsia. 1999;40 Suppl 5:S11-6.
62. Rey E, Pons G, Olive G. Vigabatrin. Clinical pharmacokinetics. Clin Pharmacokinet. 1992;23(4):267-78.
63. Curatolo P, Bombardieri R, Jozwiak S. Tuberous sclerosis. Lancet. 2008;372(9639): 657-68.
64. Hancock EC, Osborne JP, Edwards SW. Treatment of infantile spasms. Cochrane Database Syst Rev. 2013;(6):CD001770.
65. Vigabatrin Paediatric Advisory Group. Guideline for prescribing vigabatrin in children has been revised. BMJ. 2000;320(7246):1404-5.
66. Wang S, Fallah A. Optimal management of seizures associated with tuberous sclerosis complex: current and emerging options. Neuropsychiatr Dis Treat. 2014;10:2021-30.
67. French JA, Kanner AM, Bautista J, et al. Efficacy and tolerability of the new antiepileptic drugs, II: treatment of refractory epilepsy: report of the TTA and QSS Subcommittees of the American Academy of Neurology and the American Epilepsy Society. Epilepsia. 2004;45:410-23.
68. Bockbrader HN, Wesche D, Miller R, et al. A comparison of the pharmacokinetics and pharmacodynamics of pregabalin and gabapentin. Clin Pharmacokinet. 2010;49:661-9.
69. Beydoun A, Uthman BM, Kugler AR, et al. Safety and efficacy of two pregabalin regimens for add-on treatment of partial epilepsy. Neurology. 2005;64: 475-80.
70. Rogawski MA, Hanada T. Preclinical pharmacology of perampanel, a selective non-competitive AMPA receptor antagonist. Acta Neurol Scand Suppl. 2013;197: 19-24.
71. Gidal BE, Ferry J, Majid O, et al. Concentration-effect relationships with perampanel in patients with pharmacoresistant partial-onset seizures. Epilepsia. 2013;54:1490-7.
72. Treven M, Koenig X, Assadpour E, et al. The anticonvulsant retigabine is a subtype selective modulator of GABAA receptors. Epilepsia. 2015;56:647-57.

73. Faulkner MA, Burke RA. Safety profile of two novel antiepileptic agents approved for the treatment of refractory partial seizures: ezogabine (retigabine) and perampanel. Expert Opin Drug Saf. 2013;12(6):847-55.
74. Porter RJ, Partiot A, Sachdeo R, et al. Randomized, multicenter, dose-ranging trial of retigabine for partial-onset seizures. Neurology. 2007;68(15):1197-204.
75. Garin Shkolnik T, Feuerman H, Didkovsky E, et al. Blue-gray mucocutaneous discoloration: a new adverse effect of ezogabine. JAMA Dermatol. 2014;150:984-9.
76. Deeks E D. Scott LJ. Rufinamide. CNS Drugs. 2006;20:751-60.
77. Besag FM. Rufinamide for the treatment of Lennox-Gastaut syndrome. Expert Opin Pharmacother. 2011;12(5):801-6.
78. Alsaad AM, Koren G. Exposure to rufinamide and risks of CNS adverse events in drug-resistant epilepsy: a meta-analysis of randomized, placebo-controlled trials. Br J Clin Pharmacol. 2014;78:1264-71.
79. Chiron C, Marchand MC, Tran A, et al. Stiripentol in severe myoclonic epilepsy in infancy: a randomised placebo-controlled syndrome-dedicated trial. STICLO Study Group. Lancet. 2000;356:1638-42.
80. Pulman J, Hutton JL, Marson AG. Tiagabine add-on for drug-resistant partial epilepsy. Cochrane Database Syst Rev. 2014;(2):CD001908.
81. Klein P, Tyrlikova I, Brazdil M, et al. Brivaracetam for the treatment of epilepsy. Expert Opin Pharmacother. 2016;17:283-95.
82. Lattanzi S, Cagnetti C, Foschi N, et al. Brivaracetam add-on for refractory focal epilepsy: A systematic review and meta-analysis. Neurology. 2016;86(14): 1344-52.

3
CHAPTER

Older Antiepileptic Drugs

Sujit Abajirao Jagtap

INTRODUCTION

Epilepsy is most common neurological disorder affecting approximately 60 million people worldwide, with an annual incidence of 50–70 cases per 100,000 population.[1] Around 60–70% patients have focal seizures and 30–40% have seizures that are generalized at onset, including generalized onset tonic-clonic seizures, absence seizures and myoclonic seizures.[2] Most patients with generalized seizures are thought to have a genetic predisposition, the so-called genetic epilepsy. Although more than 200 antiepileptic drugs (AEDs) have been described, only a few are in common use and are called as first-generation AEDs or the standard AEDs (Table 1). These include phenytoin (PHT), phenobarbital (PB), carbamazepine (CBZ), valproic acid (VPA) and ethosuximide (ESM), which are discussed in details here with their advantages and disadvantages.

PHENOBARBITAL

Phenobarbital, the oldest AED discovered in 1912, is also known as phenobarbitone or phenobarb.

Mechanism of Action

It enhances the action of the inhibitory neurotransmitter gamma-aminobutyric acid (GABA).

Pharmacodynamics/Kinetics

Onset of action: Oral—≥60 minutes; intravenous—5 minutes.

Duration of action: Oral—10–12 hours; intravenous—>6 hours.

Absorption: Oral—rapid.

Metabolism: It is metabolized in the liver by oxidation via CYP2C9 and to a lesser extent via CYP2C19 and CYP2E1, as well as by N-glucosidation and excreted in urine (25–50% as

TABLE 1: Mechanism of action, therapeutic plasma level, half-life and dose of first-line antiepileptic drugs.

Drug	Mechanism of action	Therapeutic plasma drug concentration (µg/mL)	Half-life ($t_{1/2}$)	Maintenance dose (mg)	Principal use
Phenobarbital	Increases GABA (Fig. 1)	10–40	90 hours	60–180	Tonic-clonic, focal epilepsy
Phenytoin	Sodium channel blocker (Fig. 2)	10–20	24 hours (wide variation, dose-dependent)	300–400	Tonic-clonic, focal epilepsy
Carbamazepine	Sodium channel blocker (Fig. 2)	6–12	10–17 hours	400–1,200	Focal epilepsy, tonic-clonic
Valproic acid	Sodium channel blocker (Fig. 2) Increases GABA	50–125	15 hours	750–2,000 (20–60 mg/kg); bid-qid	Generalized epilepsy, focal epilepsy, absence seizures
Ethosuximide	Modulation of T-type calcium channels	40–100	60 hours, adult 30 hours, child	750–1,250 (20–40 mg/kg)	Absence seizures

(GABA: gamma-aminobutyric acid)

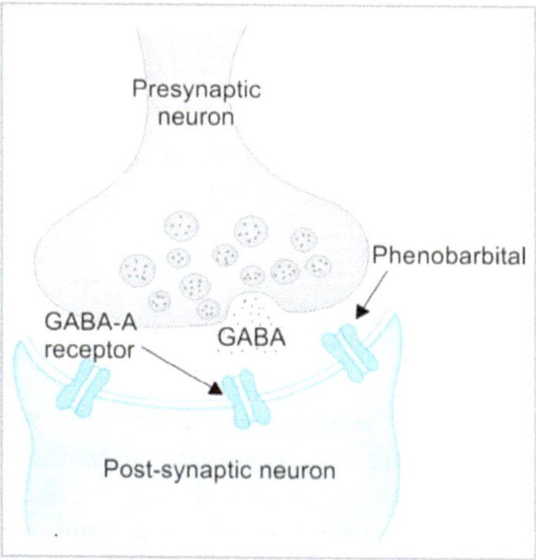

FIG. 1: Mechanism of action of phenobarbital.

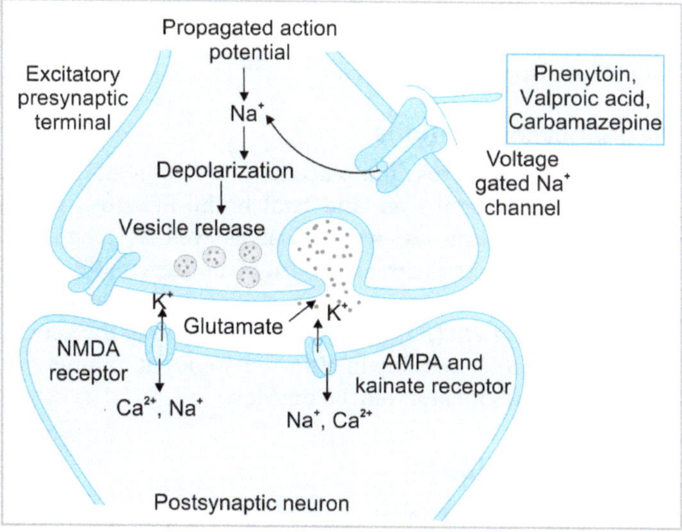

FIG. 2: Mechanism of action of phenytoin, carbamazepine and valproic acid.

unchanged drug). The elimination half-life of PB in children is ~110 hours (range: 60–180 hours) and adults is ~79 hours (range: 53–118 hours). The time to peak plasma level, by oral route, is 1.4 hours (0.5–4 hours).

Indications

It is drug of choice for the treatment of neonatal seizures and is useful for all types of seizures except for absence seizures. It is equivalent to PHT in seizure control rate; however, PHT has a better tolerability than PB. It is second-line drug in the management of status epilepticus (SE), along with PHT, when the first-line drugs (benzodiazepines) fail.[3]

Dose

Status epilepticus: Intravenous—15 mg/kg.

Maintenance dose for epilepsy (usually starts 12 hours after loading dose): Oral—60–200 mg/day or 50–100 mg two to three times daily.

Side Effects

Bradycardia, hypotension and syncope are important cardiac side effects.

Agitation, anxiety, ataxia, central nervous system (CNS) stimulation, CNS depression, confusion, dizziness, drowsiness, hallucination, hangover effect, headache, impaired judgment, insomnia, lethargy, nervousness, nightmares are major neurological side effects.

Exfoliative dermatitis, skin rash or Stevens-Johnson syndrome (SJS) are rare. Apnea (especially with rapid IV use), hypoventilation and respiratory depression can affect respiratory status. Behavioral disturbances have been frequently reported with PB as also with clonazepam.

Pregnancy Implications

Phenobarbital can cross the placenta and has been detected in the placenta, fetal liver and fetal brain. Seizures, hyperirritability, symptoms of withdrawal as well as respiratory depression may occur in the newborn of mothers on PB during pregnancy. The risk of major congenital malformation and low intelligence quotient (IQ) with PB is higher than in the general population (6.5%), possibly in a dose-dependent manner and noted with doses greater than 60 mg/day.[4]

Contraindications

Marked hepatic and renal impairment; dyspnea or airway obstruction; porphyria, hypersensitivity to PB, barbiturates or any component of the formulation.

Monitoring Parameters

Normal/therapeutic PB serum concentrations: 10–40 mg/L.

A clear correlation between serum PB concentrations and therapeutic response has not been demonstrated.

Routine monitoring—not recommended.

Drug Interactions

Phenobarbital is a cytochrome P450 (CYP450) hepatic enzyme inducer. It binds transcription factor receptors that activate CYP450 transcription, thereby increasing its amount, leading to increased activity of the CYP450 enzyme system. This results in a faster clearance of the drug metabolized by CYP450 enzyme system, reducing their duration of action and therefore their effectiveness.

Pricing: Syrup—₹45; tablets (PB oral)—30 tablets ₹48.

PHENYTOIN

Phenytoin was first made by the German chemist, Heinrich Biltz, in 1936, found to have antiepileptic properties.[5] It is better tolerated than PB.[2]

Mechanism of Action

Phenytoin limits the repetitive firing of action potentials evoked by a sustained depolarization. This effect is mediated by delaying the rate of recovery of the inactivated voltage-gated sodium channels.

Pharmacodynamics/Kinetics

Onset of action: Oral—≥60 minutes; intravenous—<30 minutes.

Duration of action: Oral—10–12 hours; intravenous—>6 hours.

Absorption: Oral—rapid.

Metabolism: Phenytoin is primarily metabolized to its inactive form by the enzyme CYP2C9. After absorption, PHT is extensively (~90%) bound to serum proteins, mainly albumin. Small variations in the bound fraction dramatically affect the absolute amount of free (active) drug. Higher proportion of free drug is evident in neonate, in patients with hypoalbuminemia, and in uremic patients.

The rate of elimination of PHT is nonlinear and varies as a function of its plasma concentration. The half-life of PHT ranges between 6 hours and 24 hours at plasma concentrations <10 µg/mL but gets prolonged with higher concentrations. As a result, plasma concentration increases disproportionately as dosage is increased, even with small adjustments near the therapeutic range. PHT is available in rapid-release and extended-release oral forms; once-daily dosing is possible only with extended-release formulations. Due to differences in dissolution and other product/formulation-dependent factors, plasma PHT level may alter with change from one formulation to the other.

Indications

It is useful for focal epilepsy as well as for generalized tonic-clonic seizures, but not absence seizures.[2] It is second-line drug in SE, after benzodiazepines fail.[4]

Seizures

- Focal seizures
- *Seizures during surgery:* Used for prevention and treatment of seizures occurring during and after neurosurgery/head injury
- *Status epilepticus:* Considered after failed treatment using a benzodiazepine due to slow onset of action[4]
- *Trigeminal neuralgia:* Drug of second choice after CBZ.[5]

Dose

Status epilepticus: Intravenous—15 mg/kg.

Maintenance dose for epilepsy (Note: maintenance dose usually starts 12 hours after loading dose): Oral—100–300 mg/day or 50–100 mg two to three times daily.

Special Considerations

- *Monitoring plasma concentrations*: Recommended due to narrow therapeutic index; anticonvulsant effect: 10–20 µg/mL
- *Liver disease*: Do not use oral loading dose. Consider a lower or decreasing the maintenance dose
- *Kidney disease*: Do not use oral loading dose. Can begin with standard maintenance dose and adjust as needed
- Intravenous (IV) use is contraindicated in patients with sinus bradycardia, SA block, second- or third-degree AV block, Stokes-Adams syndrome, or those with known hypersensitivity to PHT or any ingredient in the formulation or to other hydantoins.

Side Effects

Nausea, stomach pain, loss of appetite, hypertrichosis and gum hyperplasia due to folate deficiency are common side effects. Toxic epidermal necrolysis (TEN), bone marrow suppression, hypotension, hypersomnolence are serious side effects.[5]

Cardiovascular

Intravenous infusion should not exceed 1-3 mg/kg/min (or 50 mg/min, whichever is slower) as rapid infusion can result in severe hypotension and cardiac arrhythmia.

Neurological

Phenytoin can produce nystagmus on lateral gaze even in therapeutic doses. Diplopia, vertical nystagmus, sedation, cerebellar ataxia and tremors are seen at toxic doses.[5] Long-term use of PHT results in cerebellar atrophy, depending on the total duration of treatment rather than the dosage of medication.[5]

Hematological

Phenytoin causes megaloblastic anemia by causing a reduction in folic acid levels. PHT acts by inhibiting intestinal conjugase, which converts folate in polyglutamate form to monoglutamate form (absorbable form) leading to folate deficiency. Thrombocytopenia, agranulocytosis and aplastic anemia are rare side effects.

Pregnancy

Phenytoin is a known teratogen. "Fetal hydantoin syndrome", due to PHT use during pregnancy, consists of craniofacial anomalies (broad nasal bridge, cleft lip and palate, microcephaly) and a mild mental retardation (average IQ = 71).[6] This syndrome resembles the well-described fetal alcohol syndrome.[6] Some recommend avoiding polytherapy of AEDs and maintaining the minimal dose possible during pregnancy; however, current data do not provide specific recommendation.

Dermatological

Hypertrichosis, SJS, purple glove syndrome, rash, exfoliative dermatitis, itching and coarsening of facial features can be seen in those taking PHT.

Stevens–Johnson syndrome and TEN are serious life-threatening skin hypersensitivity reactions seen with use of PHT and associated significantly with HLA-B*1502 allele[7] which is more commonly found in Asian population, including South Asian Indians.

Immune System

Phenytoin causes drug-induced lupus, reversible immunoglobulin A (IgA) deficiency, worsening depression, suicidal ideation.[5]

Bones

Phenytoin induces hepatic metabolic enzymes, increases metabolism of vitamin D, decreasing vitamin D levels resulting in decreased bone density and increased bone fractures.

Drug Interactions

Phenytoin is an enzyme inducer and is capable of accelerating the metabolism of a range of lipid-soluble drugs including CBZ, VPA, ESM, anticoagulants, steroids and cyclosporine. Protein-binding displacement interactions with AEDs are only clinically relevant when there is concomitant enzyme inhibition, as is the case with PHT and VPA. Warfarin and trimethoprim inhibit the metabolism of phenytoin, prolong its serum half-life and result in increase in serum phenytoin levels. So, alternative AEDs should be used in patients on warfarin and trimethoprim. Allopurinol, amiodarone, cimetidine, imipramine and some sulfonamides also inhibit the metabolism of phenytoin.

Fosphenytoin, a water-soluble prodrug of phenytoin, is rapidly converted into phenytoin by phosphatases in liver and erythrocytes. Fosphenytoin is extensively (95–99%) bound to plasma proteins, primarily albumin. This binding is saturable, and fosphenytoin can displace phenytoin from the protein-binding sites. Fosphenytoin is useful for adults with partial or generalized seizures when IV or intramuscular administration is indicated, underscoring the importance of attention to this interaction.

VALPROIC ACID

In 1963, the anticonvulsant properties of VPA were discovered serendipitously by Pierre Eymard.[5]

Mechanism of Action

Valproic acid inhibits sustained repetitive firing, induced by depolarization, by prolonging the recovery phase of voltage-activated sodium channels. VPA also reduces the T-type calcium current limiting sustained repetitive firing. Another mechanism of action of VPA involves GABA metabolism by stimulating the activity of glutamic acid decarboxylase, the GABA synthetic enzyme, and inhibiting GABA degradative enzymes.[5]

Pharmacokinetic Properties

Valproic acid is absorbed rapidly and completely after oral administration. Peak concentration in plasma is attained in 1–4 hours, or several hours later if the drug is administered in enteric-coated tablets or ingested with meals. Its extent of binding to plasma proteins is usually ~90%, but the bound fraction is reduced as the total concentration of VPA is increased through the therapeutic range.

Valproic acid (95%) undergoes hepatic metabolism [via uridine diphosphate glucuronosyltransferases (UGTs) and β-oxidation], with <5% excreted unchanged in urine. VPA is a substrate for CYP2C9 and CYP2C19, but metabolism by these enzymes accounts for a relatively minor portion of its elimination. The half-life of VPA is ~15 hours but is reduced in patients taking other AEDs.[5]

Plasma Drug Concentrations

Therapeutic effects of VPA are seen with plasma levels ranging from 30 to 100 mg/mL, but there is a poor correlation between the plasma concentration and efficacy of drug. There appears to be a threshold of plasma concentration at ~30–50 mg/mL, beyond which the plasma albumin binding sites approach saturation.

Drug Interactions

Valproic acid inhibits the metabolism of drugs that are substrates for CYP2C9, including phenytoin and PB. VPA also inhibits UGT and thus inhibits the metabolism of lamotrigine and lorazepam. VPA is highly bound to albumin and can displace phenytoin and other drugs: this displacement can exacerbate the VPA induced inhibition of phenytoin metabolism. The concurrent administration of valproate and clonazepam rarely has been associated with the development of absence SE.

Indications

Valproate is drug of choice in the treatment of absence epilepsy and juvenile myoclonic epilepsy. It is also useful in partial and tonic-clonic seizures.

The initial daily dose usually is 15 mg/kg, increased at weekly intervals by 5–10 mg/kg/day to a maximum daily dose of 60 mg/kg.

Side Effects

The most common side effects are transient gastrointestinal (GI) symptoms, including anorexia, nausea and vomiting in ~16% of patients. CNS effects include sedation, ataxia and tremor; occur infrequently and usually respond to a decrease in dosage. Hirsutism and weight gain have been seen with chronic VPA treatment. Asymptomatic elevation of hepatic transaminases is observed in up to 40% of patients during the first several months of therapy. Fulminant hepatitis is seen rarely in children under 2 years of age, especially in those on multiple AEDs. Acute pancreatitis and hyperammonemia are also seen with the use of VPA.[5]

ETHOSUXIMIDE

The mechanism of action of succinimides is through modulation of thalamic T-type calcium currents, which block synchronized firing of neurons associated with spike and wave discharges (Fig. 3). Succinimides are absorbed orally, reaching peak concentrations within 3–7 hours. The volume of distribution is 0.6–0.7 L/kg. There is no significant protein binding. ESM is metabolized in the liver to inactive metabolite. The half-life of ESM is approximately 60 hours in adults and

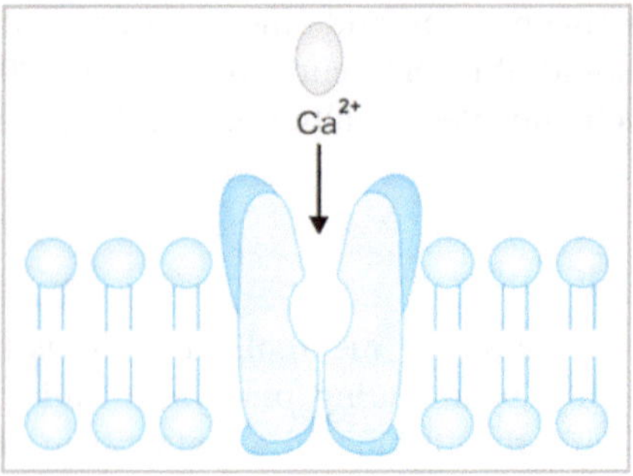

FIG. 3: Mechanism of action of ethosuximide (Inhibition of 'T' type Ca^{2+} current).

30 hours in children. ESM reaches plasma steady state level after 4–7 days of oral administration.[8] In contrast, it takes 8–16 days for the active metabolite of methsuximide to reach steady state.

Enzyme-inducing AEDs decrease the half-life of succinimides.

Indications

Ethosuximide is the drug of first choice in the treatment of absence seizures, a form of primary generalized epilepsy. ESM, in combination with VPA, may also be effective for myoclonic absence seizures.[8]

Dose

The starting dose of ESM is 500 mg/day in patients above 6 years of age and is increased by 250 mg/week in adults up to maintenance doses of 1,000–2,000 mg/day. The dose for children between 3 years and 6 years of age is 10 mg/kg/day and is increased by 5–10 mg/kg/day to reach a maintenance dose of 15–40 mg/kg/day in children. ESM should be given in two to three divided doses; however, single daily doses can also be used. Dose adjustments are not needed with hepatic or renal impairment. ESM is available in 250 mg capsules and a 250 mg/5 mL.

Side Effects

The dose-related side effects of the succinimides include sedation, dizziness and headache; however, these are minor. Movement disorders and psychosis are unusual CNS side effects associated with succinimides. More commonly, gastric side effects limit the use of succinimides. This includes gastric upset, anorexia, nausea and vomiting. Taking these medications after meals can minimize these symptoms. Idiosyncratic reactions include rash and leukopenia. Rare cases of agranulocytosis, aplastic anemia and systemic lupus erythematosus have been associated with the use of succinimides.[9]

CARBAMAZEPINE

Carbamazepine was discovered in 1953 by Swiss chemist Walter Schindler.

Mechanism of Action

Carbamazepine is a sodium channel blocker and acts by binding to inactivated voltage-gated sodium channels and thereby preventing repetitive and sustained firing of an action potential.[5,10]

Pharmacokinetic Properties

Onset of action: Oral—4.5 hours for immediate-release tablets, 3–12 hours for extended-release tablets and 1.5 hours for oral suspension.

Duration of action: About 2–3 days.

Carbamazepine is absorbed well but slowly after oral administration. The plasma half-life of CBZ varies from 30 hours (when given as single dose) to about 15 hours (when given in multiple doses) as it is potent hepatic enzyme inducer and induces its own metabolism also.

Carbamazepine is almost completely metabolized in the liver mainly by CYP3A4, although CYP2C8 and CYP3A5 also play a role and only 5% of drug is excreted unchanged. It is mainly excreted in urine (72%) and rest by feces (28%). In the blood, CBZ is about 75% bound to plasma proteins. Plasma level can vary from 0.5 to 25 µg/mL and has no apparent relationship to daily drug doses. CBZ is a hepatic enzyme inducer and causes upregulation of genes involved in its own metabolism. This phenomenon is called as autoinduction and is completed after 3–5 weeks of daily dosing regimen. Drug-drug interactions through hepatic CYP3A4 enzyme system can alter CBZ plasma levels in polytherapy.[11,12]

Indications

Carbamazepine is commonly used for the treatment of epilepsy (including focal onset seizures, generalized tonic-clonic seizures and mixed seizures) as well as for neuropathic pain. It is also used in certain psychiatric disorders like bipolar disorder and in some cases of schizophrenia if treatments with conventional antipsychotics have failed alone. It is not effective for absence seizures or myoclonic seizures.[5]

Dose

Oral: 10–20 mg/kg/day bid or tid as tablets, or qid as suspension.

Adults: 400–1,200 mg.

Maintenance dose range: 800–1,200 mg/day in divided doses. Maximum dose of 1,600 mg/day recommended.

Start with 200 mg twice daily and increase weekly by 200 mg/day (up to a maximum of 1,600 mg/day) given in three or four divided doses (for regular release tablet) or in two divided doses (for extended-release tablets).

Side Effects[13,14]

Most commonly encountered side effects are dizziness, drowsiness, unsteadiness, headaches and migraines, nausea, vomiting, and/or constipation especially in the beginning of therapy which can be reduced by starting at lowest recommended dosage. Less commonly encountered adverse effects include increased risk of seizures, especially with abrupt cessation of drug and in those with mixed seizure disorders, cardiac arrhythmias and blurring of vision or diplopia.[5]

Hemopoietic System

Bone marrow depression, aplastic anemia, agranulocytosis, pancytopenia, thrombocytopenia, leukopenia, leukocytosis, eosinophilia; should be avoided in patients with history of hepatic porphyria (e.g. acute intermittent porphyria, variegate porphyria, porphyria cutanea tarda) as it can precipitate acute attacks.

Skin

Toxic epidermal necrolysis and SJS with an estimated risk of about 1–6 per 10,000 new users of CBZ among Caucasian populations and 10 times higher risk in some Asian countries. This risk is related to high prevalence of HLA-B*1502 in Asians, which predisposes to severe drug-induced skin reactions. It is recommended that prior to starting CBZ therapy, HLA-B*1502 testing should be done in patients of such ancestry wherein there is high prevalence of the allele. CBZ should be discontinued at the first sign of a rash and replaced with an alternative AED. The HLA-B*1502 allele, however, does not predict risk of less severe adverse cutaneous reactions.[15]

Cardiovascular System

Congestive heart failure, aggravation of hypertension, hypotension, syncope, collapse, aggravation of coronary artery disease, arrhythmias and AV block, thrombophlebitis, thromboembolism (e.g. pulmonary embolism) and lymphadenopathy. Cardiovascular complications can be fatal. Myocardial infarction has been associated with other tricyclic compounds.

Liver

Deranged liver function test (LFT), jaundice (both cholestatic and hepatocellular), hepatitis, very rare cases of hepatic failure; hypercholesterolemia.

Genitourinary System

Increased frequency, acute retention of urine, acute renal failure with oliguria, elevated blood urea and high blood pressure (BP); also impotence and rarely impaired male fertility.

Digestive System

Loss of appetite, nausea, vomiting, gastric irritation and pain abdomen; diarrhea as well as constipation, loss of appetite, dry mouth and glossitis.

Metabolism

Hyponatremia and risk of syndrome of inappropriate secretion of antidiuretic hormone (SIADH) (BOXED WARNINGS). Risk of osteoporosis is due to decreased calcium levels.

Contraindications

- Atonic seizures, myoclonic seizures, absence seizures
- Hypersensitivity to barbiturates, CBZ, hydantoin or tricyclic antidepressant
- Renal failure or impairment
- Geriatric—more susceptible to CNS and cardiac side effects as well as SIADH
- Pregnancy—teratogenic; causes congenital malformations, including spina bifida, craniofacial defects and cardiovascular malformations; also leads to developmental delay. Neonates can develop withdrawal syndrome if used during pregnancy
- Breastfeeding—due to risk of adverse effect (especially hepatitis)
- Monoamine oxidase inhibitor (MAOI) therapy—contraindicated in patients on MAOI therapy.

Drug Concentration

Routine periodic monitoring of serum CBZ concentrations is recommended.

Drug Interactions

Phenytoin, PB or primidone lower blood levels of CBZ; can lead to seizure precipitation. Being a potent inducer of CYP450 enzyme, CBZ itself enhances clearance of many drugs, leading to decreased blood levels and reduced activity. The drugs metabolized by CBZ include warfarin, lamotrigine, phenytoin, theophylline, VPA, benzodiazepines and oral contraceptive pills. Some drugs decrease the rate of metabolism of CBZ and thus increase the blood, which include erythromycin, cimetidine, propoxyphene and calcium channel blockers and VPA.

REFERENCES

1. Hauser WA, Annegers JF, Rocca WA. Descriptive epidemiology of epilepsy: contributions of population-based studies from Rochester, Minnesota. Mayo Clin Proc. 1996;71:576-86.
2. Chadwick DW. Diagnosis of epilepsy. Lancet. 1990;336:291-5.
3. Brodie MJ, Kwan P. Current position of phenobarbital in epilepsy and its future. Epilepsia. 2012;53 (Suppl 8):40-6.
4. Glauser T, Shinnar S, Gloss D, et al. Evidence-based guideline: treatment of convulsive status epilepticus in children and adults: report of the Guideline Committee of the American Epilepsy Society. Epilepsy Curr. 2016;16(1):48-61.
5. Hardman JG, Limbird LE, Gilman AG. Goodman and Gilman's: The Pharmacological Basis of Therapeutics, 10th edition. New York: McGraw-Hill. 2001.
6. Harden CL, Pennell PB, Koppel BS, et al. Practice parameter update: management issues for women with epilepsy—focus on pregnancy (an evidence-based review): vitamin K, folic acid, blood levels, and breastfeeding: report of the Quality Standards Subcommittee and Therapeutics and Technology Assessment Subcommittee of the American Academy of Neurology and American Epilepsy Society. Neurology. 2009;73(2):142-9.
7. Man CB, Kwan P, Baum L, et al. Association between HLA-B*1502 allele and antiepileptic drug-induced cutaneous reactions in Han Chinese. Epilepsia. 2007;48(5):1015-8.
8. Glauser TA, Cnaan A, Shinnar S, et al. Ethosuximide, valproic acid, and lamotrigine in childhood absence epilepsy. N Engl J Med. 2010;362(9):790-9.
9. Vajda FJ, Eadie MJ. The clinical pharmacology of traditional antiepileptic drugs. Epileptic Disord. 2014;16(4):395-408.
10. Flynn S, Babi MA. Anticonvulsants. In: Dowd FJ, Johnson BS, Mariotti AJ (Eds). Pharmacology and Therapeutics for Dentistry, 7th edition. St. Louis: Elsevier; 2017. p. 176.
11. Bentley P, Sharma P. Neurological disorders—epilepsy, Parkinson's disease and multiple sclerosis. In: Bennett PN, Brown MJ, Sharma P (Eds). Clinical Pharmacology, 11th edition. Edinburgh: Churchill Livingstone; 2012.
12. Cotterman-Hart S. Antiepileptic drugs: first generation. In: Newton HB, Maschio M (Eds). Epilepsy and Brain Tumors; Amsterdam: Elsevier; 2015. pp. 159-69.
13. Pellock JM. Carbamazepine side effects in children and adults. Epilepsia. 1987;28 (Suppl 3):S64-70.
14. Keränen T, Sivenius J. Side effects of carbamazepine, valproate and clonazepam during long-term treatment of epilepsy. Acta Neurol Scand Suppl. 1983;97:69-80.
15. Lim KS, Kwan P, Tan CT. Association of HLA-B*1502 allele and carbamazepine-induced severe adverse cutaneous drug reaction among Asians, a review. Neurology Asia. 2008;13:15-21.

4 CHAPTER

Newer Antiepileptic Drugs

Neeraj N Baheti

INTRODUCTION

Antiepileptic drug (AED) selection is based on efficacy in the given epilepsy syndrome and patient-specific factors including comorbidities. Over the last two decades, more than 16 newer AEDs acting on different receptors (Table 1) have been approved and marketed. Given such a large number of newer AEDs available, a thorough knowledge of efficacy, pharmacokinetic properties, drug interactions, safety and tolerability profile, and its efficacy against comorbidities is of utmost importance while selecting AED specific to the patient's circumstances. The AEDs are discussed focusing on mechanism of action, pharmacokinetics, drug interactions, approved indications, adverse effects, and dosing and administration. The third-generation AEDs are covered in a separate chapter.

OXCARBAZEPINE

Oxcarbazepine is the 10-keto analog of carbamazepine (CBZ), which blocks high frequency voltage-dependent repetitive neuronal firing of sodium channels (Fig. 1).[1] Oxcarbazepine (OXC) has excellent oral bioavailability and low protein binding. After absorption, it is rapidly converted to monohydroxy derivative (MHD) licarbazepine, which is responsible for antiseizure activity. The half-life of active MHD is 8–10 hours, unlike CBZ no autoinduction is seen on chronic therapy. OXC is metabolized in the liver. It is a weak inducer of CYP3A4 and reduces the efficacy of the oral contraceptive pill at high doses (>900 mg). It is a weak inhibitor of CYP2C19, thus raising the levels of phenytoin (PHT) and phenobarbitone especially when used at high doses.[2]

Indication

Oxcarbazepine is approved as a first-line therapy for focal and secondarily generalized seizures in children and adults. It may

TABLE 1: Mechanism of action of newer antiepileptic drugs.

Drug	Sodium channels	Calcium channels	Potassium channels	Enhancing GABA	Inhibiting glutamate	SV2A binding	Remarks
Brivaracetam						++	
Clobazam				++			
Gabapentin	+	+		++			
Lacosamide	++						Selective slow voltage-gated sodium channels
Lamotrigine	++	+					
Levetiracetam		+	+	+	+	++	
Oxcarbazepine	++	+	+				
Perampanel					++		Noncompetitive AMPA receptor
Rufinamide	++						
Topiramate	+	+		+	++		Kainate, AMPA and CA receptor antagonist
Zonisamide	+	+					

(+: minor action; ++: major action; AMPA: α-amino-3-hydroxy-5-methyl-4-isoxazole-propionic acid; CA: carbonic anhydrase; GABA: gamma aminobutyric acid; SV2A: synaptic vesicle protein 2A)

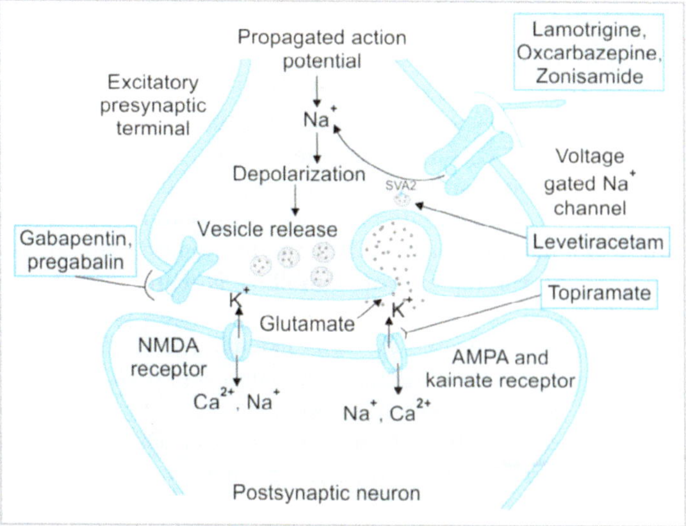

FIG. 1: Mechanism of action of various newer antiepileptic drugs.

exacerbate absence and myoclonic seizures, hence it better avoided in patients with generalized epilepsy.[3,4]

Clinical Implications

Oxcarbazepine with lesser drug interactions, better pharmacokinetics and better safety profile (no epoxy derivative, no autoinduction) is a good alternative first line therapy for focal onset seizures especially in children. It may be particularly useful in patients who respond to CBZ but are unable to tolerate due to adverse effects. However, it is far costlier than CBZ.

Side Effects

Sedation, headache, fatigue, dizziness, blurred vision, diplopia, nausea, vomiting and ataxia are the most commonly reported adverse effects. Rash may occur in 2–4% of individuals. Around 25% of individuals who experience rash with CBZ may also experience it with OXC. OXC is more likely to cause hyponatremia than CBZ especially in older individuals and those taking a diuretic. Very rarely cases of agranulocytosis, aplastic anemia, pancytopenia and thrombocytopenia have been reported with OXC.

Dosage and Administration

Oxcarbazepine is only available as an oral preparation. OXC can be started with initial dose of 300 mg (5–8 mg/kg/day) in two divided doses increasing by 300 mg every week up to a maximum of 1,200 mg twice daily (30 mg/kg/day). Conversion from CBZ can be done overnight; the dose needs to be 1.5 times the CBZ dose.[1]

LAMOTRIGINE

It acts by blocking the voltage-dependent sodium channels (Fig. 1). There is some evidence that it also inhibits the release of glutamate through stabilization of presynaptic membrane. Lamotrigine (LTG) has an excellent oral bioavailability and it is 55% protein bound. It is metabolized in the liver, predominantly by glucuronidation and then eliminated in the urine. The half-life is about 24 hours in monotherapy. In the presence of valproate, which inhibits glucuronidation the half-life is doubled and drug levels can markedly increase.[5] In the presence of enzyme inducers like CBZ, PHT, rifampicin, the plasma half-life is reduced by half. Combined estrogen-progestin contraceptives decrease LTG levels by increasing clearance conversely; LTG may reduce the effectiveness of combined estrogen-progestin contraceptives.

Dosage and Administration

Lamotrigine is available as an oral preparation only. LTG requires a very slow titration to avoid the development of rash. In monotherapy, start as 25 mg/day for 2 weeks, hike to 50 mg/day for another 2 weeks; thereafter the dose is increased by 50 mg every 1–2 weeks until an optimum response is achieved. The titration rate is half as fast with adjunctive valproic acid, but can be twice as fast in the presence of enzyme inducers.[6] The usual maintenance dose is 200–500 mg and in the presence of concomitant valproate restricted to 100–300 mg. The suggested therapeutic range is 2–20 mg/L. It is also available as extended-release preparation allowing once-daily dosing and also reducing toxicity from peak levels. LTG clearance increases by approximately 65% in pregnancy thus frequent monitoring and dose adjustment is recommended.[7]

Indication

Lamotrigine is approved by FDA for the adjunctive treatment of focal seizures, generalized tonic-clonic seizures and Lennox–Gastaut syndrome (LGS).[4] LTG is a recommended first-line AED for focal seizures and generalized tonic-clonic seizures.[5] Although recommended in generalized absence seizures also but it is less effective than valproate and ethosuximide. It may be effective against myoclonic seizures in some patients, but may exacerbate these seizures in others.[8]

Clinical Implications

Lamotrigine is an effective broad-spectrum AED for the treatment of all types of seizures except myoclonic jerks. In polytherapy, LTG is particularly efficacious with valproate and this combination may be ideal for drug-resistant generalized epilepsies including those with myoclonic jerks. Usually, small doses of LTG added to valproate may render previously intractable patients seizure free. In view of mood stabilizing property, it can be a good choice of AED in patients with comorbid mood disorders.

Side Effects

Common dose related side effects include sedation, dizziness, diplopia, ataxia, nausea, vomiting and tremors. Serious side effects of LTG often requiring drug withdrawals include skin rash and rarely Steven-Johnson syndrome and toxic epidermal necrolysis. The risk of rash increases when LTG is administered with valproate or when the dose is titrated rapidly.[9]

TOPIRAMATE

Topiramate (TPM) has multiple mechanisms of action. It enhances gamma-aminobutyric acid (GABA) mediated inhibition, blocks voltage-dependent sodium channels and L-type voltage-activated calcium channels and antagonizes N-methyl-D-aspartate (NMDA)-glutamate receptor (Fig. 1). It is also a weak inhibitor of carbonic anhydrase. TPM has an excellent oral bioavailability (>80%). Its protein binding is not clinically significant. It is partially metabolized in the liver and about 70% is eliminated unchanged in the urine. Its half-life is approximately 20–30 hours when used as monotherapy. Enzyme-inducing AEDs can reduce plasma levels of TPM by nearly half by increasing clearance. Conversely, TPM can reduce PHT clearance thus increasing blood levels. TPM may reduce the effectiveness of hormonal contraceptives.[2]

Dosage and Administration

Topiramate is available as oral preparation only. TPM is initiated at 25 mg twice daily, the dose can be increased by 25–50 mg every week. The dose can be hiked up to 200–400 mg/day and in the presence of enzyme-inducing AEDs, the dose can be hiked up to 600 mg/day.

Indication

Topiramate is a broad-spectrum AED. TPM is approved as monotherapy or adjunctive therapy for focal and generalized tonic-clonic seizures in patients 2 years and elders.[4] It is approved for adjunctive treatment of seizures associated with LGS.[10] Although approved, TPM is usually not preferred as first line because of its cognitive adverse effects, unless its use is justified by comorbidity such as migraine or obesity.[11]

Clinical Implications

Topiramate is a broad-spectrum AED useful in as adjuvant therapy in resistant focal and symptomatic generalized epilepsies. It can be preferred as initial monotherapy in obese or with concomitant migraine.

Side Effects

Common adverse effects include psychomotor slowing, decreased attention, executive dysfunction, impairment of language, word-finding difficulty, reduced verbal fluency and slurred speech. Other side effects include sedation, fatigue, dizziness, ataxia and depression. In children, hypohydrosis, hyperthermia and metabolic acidosis are rare serious side effects. Acute myopia, secondary angle glaucoma and renal stones have also been reported. Weight loss is a common dose-related side effect. Paresthesia of hands and feet is another commonly reported adverse effect probably related to carbonic anhydrase inhibition. Hyperammonemia may occur, especially, if used in conjunction with valproate.[12]

CLOBAZAM

Clobazam is 1,5-benzodiazepine, enhances the inhibitory effects of GABA. It binds to the GABA-A receptor and increases the frequency of GABA-mediated chloride channel openings.[13] Clobazam has good oral bioavailability and is highly protein bound (85%). Clobazam is metabolized in the liver to the active N-desmethylclobazam. Elimination half-life in adults is 10–30 hours, justifying once daily dosing. Dose adjustments are required in patients with hepatic insufficiency. Enzyme-inducing AEDs can increase plasma clearance of clobazam and decrease serum levels.

Dosage and Administration

Clobazam is available as oral preparation only. Clobazam is usually initiated at 5 mg/day in one dose, typically given at bedtime. The dose may be increased every 1–2 weeks to a maximum of 40 mg/day. Unlike other benzodiazepines, clobazam has least propensity for tolerance.

Indication

Clobazam is a broad spectrum AED used as an adjunctive therapy in focal and generalized tonic-clonic seizures especially in drug-resistant epilepsy scenarios. In United States, clobazam is recently approved as an adjunctive therapy in LGS.[14]

Clinical Implications

Clobazam is a broad spectrum, good adjunctive medication useful in all drug-resistant epilepsies. It has a lower propensity for tolerance and drug dependence compared to other benzodiazepines. It is a very good add-on drug for focal epilepsy and can be used for long-term.

Side Effects

Adverse effects include somnolence and sedation, dysarthria, drooling, aggression or other behavioral changes. Withdrawal seizures may occur with abrupt discontinuation.

LEVETIRACETAM

Levetiracetam (LEV) acts by novel mechanisms by inhibiting the synaptic vesicle protein SV2A, an integral membrane glycoprotein involved in synaptic vesicle exocytosis (Fig. 1).[15] There is also evidence that LEV indirectly modulates GABA and glycine gated currents, and can partially inhibit N-type calcium.[16] LEV has an excellent oral bioavailability (95%) and very low protein binding. It has no hepatic metabolism; 66% is excreted unchanged in the urine and the rest is hydrolyzed to inactive compounds. The half-life is 6–8 hours in adults. It has no known significant pharmacokinetic interactions.

Indications

Levetiracetam is a broad-spectrum drug, approved as an adjunctive therapy for focal onset seizures, generalized tonic-clonic seizures, and generalized myoclonic seizures.[4] Intravenous preparation has shown efficacy in acute seizures and status epilepticus.

Clinical Implications

Levetiracetam is a broad-spectrum drug with a favorable pharmacokinetic profile in terms of safety and absence of any interactions with other AEDs or concomitant medications. It is a first line contender for idiopathic generalized epilepsy where it is replacing valproate and in focal seizures where it is a main challenger for CBZ, especially in child-bearing age group females.

Adverse Effects

Levetiracetam is usually well tolerated. The most common adverse effects include headache, dizziness, asthenia and somnolence. A reversible thrombocytopenia is seen in a small number of patients. However, there are concerns of behavioral side effects like aggression, emotional labiality, oppositional behavior and psychosis especially in children or those who are intellectually disabled and have baseline behavioral problems.[17,18]

Dosage and Administration

Levetiracetam is available in oral and intravenous formulations. Initiate levetiracetam as 500 mg (10 mg/kg/day) in two divided doses. The dose can be hiked every 2 weeks as needed for seizure control. Usual maintenance dose is 2,000–3,000 mg/day; some patients may tolerate and respond to doses as high as 4,000 mg/day. In children usual maintenance dose is 30–40 mg/kg; doses up to 60 mg/kg/day may be needed and well tolerated by younger children.

ZONISAMIDE

Zonisamide is structurally a sulfonamide derivative, which has multiple mechanisms of action. It acts by blocking sodium channels, T-type calcium channels and carbonic anhydrase inhibition (Fig. 1). Zonisamide has excellent oral bioavailability (>90%) and low protein binding (40%). It is metabolized primarily in the liver and excreted through kidney. It has a long half-life of around 60 hours. It is not recommended in patients with severe hepatic or renal impairment. It is not an enzyme inducer or inhibitor but its clearance may be increased when used enzyme-inducing AEDs like CBZ, PHT or phenobarbital.

Indication

Zonisamide is a broad-spectrum agent approved as an adjuvant therapy for focal seizures in adults and children.[19,20] It has also been approved as monotherapy for focal seizures in Europe and generalized epilepsy in Japan.

Clinical Implications

Zonisamide is an effective broad-spectrum AED useful as an adjunctive therapy in drug-resistant epilepsy and epileptic encephalopathies. It is quite effective in myoclonic jerks and hence can be used is idiopathic generalized epilepsies.

Dosage and Administration

The starting dose is 100–200 mg/day for 2 weeks. Because of its long half-life, once-a-day dosing is often effective. The dose can be increased by 100 mg every 2 weeks up to 600 mg/day as needed for seizure control.

Side Effects

Most common adverse effects include somnolence, ataxia, anorexia, weight loss and agitation or irritability. Other rare side effects include severe skin rash like Stevens-Johnson syndrome or toxic epidermal necrolyisis. It can lead to oligohydrosis, hyperthermia and nephrolithiasis especially in children. Cognitive slowing and difficulty with concentration may be seen, particularly at higher doses.

GABAPENTIN

Gabapentin binds to the α2-δ subunit of voltage-gated calcium channels, reducing the influx of calcium and associated neurotransmitter release, thus in turn decreasing excitablity (Fig. 1).[21] Gabapentin is absorbed by means of saturable amino acid transport systems in the gut and the bioavailability of gabapentin is low (<60%). The drug does not bind to plasma protein, nor is it metabolized. It is eliminated unchanged in the urine. Its half-life is 5-7 hours. It has no known interactions, other than potential antacid interference with its absorption.[22]

Dosage and Administration

The recommended starting dose of gabapentin is 300–400 mg/day, increased by 300-400 mg every day up to 300-400 mg three times a day. The dose can be increased as needed up to 3,600 mg/day in three divided doses. The antiseizure effects of gabapentin are dose related, and the therapeutic effects of doses less than 900 mg/day may be small.

Indication

Gabapentin is approved as monotherapy or adjunctive therapy for focal seizures with or without secondary generalization.[4] Although approved in Europe for initial monotherapy, a large randomized comparative trial found it less effective than LTG.[5]

Clinical Implications

Gabapentin appears to be a narrow-spectrum AED whose role in the management of partial seizures is limited because its efficacy is weak compared with other AEDs.

Side Effects

The common adverse effects include drowsiness, dizziness, ataxia, tiredness and weight gain. It may cause cognitive slowing in the elderly and emotional labiality in children.

PREGABALIN

Pregabalin modulates $\alpha 2$-δ protein subunit of voltage-gated calcium channels reducing calcium influx and excitability (Fig. 1).[21]

It does not bind to plasma proteins. The elimination half-life is 5–7 hours, it is excreted unchanged in urine. It has no significant interactions with other drugs.

Dosage and Administration

The starting dose is 75 mg once (at bedtime) or twice daily. The dose can be increased by 75 mg every week as needed, until seizure control, appearance of adverse effects, or reaching a maximum dose of 300 mg two times a day.

Indication

Pregabalin is a narrow-spectrum drug against focal seizures. The official FDA epilepsy indication is adjunctive therapy for adult patients with focal onset seizures.[4] Pregabalin may exacerbate generalized myoclonic and absence seizures.[23]

Clinical Implications

Although approved as adjunctive therapy, the role of pregabalin in management of partial seizures is not fully ascertained. It is reserved for intractable partial seizures who have failed to respond to other AED combinations.

Side Effects

The most common side effects include dizziness, somnolence, increased appetite, weight gain and peripheral edema.

CONCLUSION

Many newer and safer AEDs are available for the treatment of epilepsy. The knowledge of pharmacokinetics, efficacy and tolerability profiles facilitates the choice of appropriate antiepileptic medication for patients with epilepsy.

REFERENCES

1. Bang LM, Goa KL. Spotlight on oxcarbazepine in epilepsy. CNS Drugs. 2004;18(1):57-61.
2. Johannessen LC, Patsalos PN. Drug interactions involving the new second- and third-generation antiepileptic drugs. Expert Rev. Neurother. 2010;10:119-40.
3. Gelisse P, Genton P, Kuate D, et al. Worsening of seizures by oxcarbazepine in juvenile idiopathic generalized epilepsies. Epilepsia. 2004;45(10):1282-8.
4. Food and Drug Administration (FDA). FDA labelling information. [online] Available from http://www.accessdata.fda.gov/scripts/cder/drugsatfda/index.cfm. [Last accessed June 2019].

5. Marson AG, Al-Kharusi AM, Alwaidh M, et al. The SANAD study of effectiveness of carbamazepine, gabapentin, lamotrigine, oxcarbazepine, or topiramate for treatment of partial epilepsy: an unblinded randomised controlled trial. Lancet. 2007;369(9566):1000-15.
6. Brigo F, Ausserer H, Tezzon F, et al. When one plus one makes three: the quest for rational antiepileptic polytherapy with supraadditive anticonvulsant efficacy. Epilepsy Behav. 2013;27(3):439-42.
7. Patsalos PN, Berry DJ, Bourgeois BF, et al. Antiepileptic drugs–Best practice guidelines for therapeutic drug monitoring: a position paper by the Subcommission on Therapeutic Drug Monitoring, ILAE Commission on Therapeutic Strategies. Epilepsia. 2008;49(7):1239-76.
8. Barron TF, Hunt SL, Hoban TF, et al. Lamotrigine monotherapy in children. Pediatric Neurology. 2000;23(2):160-3.
9. Guberman AH, Besag FM, Brodie MJ, et al. Lamotrigine- associated rash: risk/benefit considerations in adults and children. Epilepsia. 1999;40(7):985-91.
10. Sachdeo RC, Glauser TA, Ritter F, et al. A double-blind, randomized trial of topiramate in Lennox-Gastaut syndrome. Neurology. 1999;52(9):1882-7.
11. Meador KJ, Loring DW, Hulihan JF, et al; CAPSS-027 Study Group. Differential cognitive and behavioral effects of topiramate and valproate. Neurology. 2003;60(9):1483-8.
12. Hamer HM, Knake S, Schomburg U, et al. Valproate-induced hyperammonemic encephalopathy in the presence of topiramate. Neurology. 2000;54(1):230-2.
13. Ng YT, Collins SD. Clobazam. Neurotherapeutics 2007;4(1):138-44.
14. Ng YT, Conry JA, Drummond R, et al. Randomized, phase III study results of clobazam in Lennox-Gastaut syndrome. Neurology. 2011;77(15):1473-81.
15. Lynch BA, Lambeng N, Nocka K, et al. The synaptic vesicle protein SV2A is the binding site for the antiepileptic drug levetiracetam. Proc Natl Acad Sci U S A. 2004;101(26):9861-6.
16. Meehan AL, Yang X, Yuan LL, et al. Levetiracetam has an activity-dependent effect on inhibitory transmission. Epilepsia. 2012;53(3):469-76.
17. Hurtado B, Koepp MJ, Sander JW, et al. The impact of levetiracetam on challenging behavior. Epilepsy Behav. 2006;8(3):588-92.
18. Kossoff EH, Bergey GK, Freeman JM, et al. Levetiracetam psychosis in children with epilepsy. Epilepsia. 2001;42(12):1611-3.
19. Faught E, Ayala R, Montouris GG, et al. Randomized controlled trial of zonisamide for the treatment of refractory partial-onset seizures. Neurology. 2001;57(10):1774-9.
20. Glauser TA, Pellock JM. Zonisamide in pediatric epilepsy: review of the Japanese experience. J Child Neurol. 2002;17(2):87-96.
21. Fink K, Dooley DJ, Meder WP, et al. Inhibition of neuronal Ca(2+) influx by gabapentin and pregabalin in the human neocortex. Neuropharmacology. 2002;42(2):229-36.
22. Gidal BE, Radulovic LL, Kruger S, et al. Inter- and intra-subject variability in gabapentin absorption and absolute bioavailability. Epilepsy Res. 2000;40(2-3):123-7.
23. Ben-Menachem E. Pregabalin pharmacology and its relevance to clinical practice. Epilepsia. 2004;45(Suppl 6):13-18.

5

CHAPTER

Third-generation Antiepileptic Drugs

Karan M Desai, Sangeeta H Ravat

INTRODUCTION

In spite of the multitude of antiepileptic drugs (AEDs) available on the market, approximately 30% of epilepsy patients remain refractory and inadequately controlled with the current frontline AEDs.[1] For these patients, the most appropriate therapeutic option is presumably the combined administration of two or more AEDs or the application of novel AEDs. The third-generation AEDs consist of as many as 20 novel drugs some of which have novel actions.[2] For the sake of this chapter we will limit the discussion to six drugs namely perampanel (PER), brivaracetam (BRV), lacosamide (LCM), eslicarbazepine (ESL), stiripentol and rufinamide. The aim of this review is to summarize our knowledge on the current clinical status of some selected third-generation AEDs and highlight the clinically relevant points.

PERAMPANEL

Perampanel is a noncompetitive α-amino-3-hydroxy-5-methyl-4-isoxazole-propionic acid (AMPA)-type glutamate receptor antagonist. The mechanism of action of perampanel is discussed in Figure 1. It inhibits AMPA induced increases in intracellular calcium thus reducing neuronal excitability.[3] PER is available as oral formulation only. It has excellent oral bioavailability and is 95% protein-bound. It is extensively metabolized in the liver. It has a long half-life of about 105 hours. Dose adjustments are recommended for patients with mild and moderate hepatic impairment and the drug is not recommended for patients with severe hepatic or renal impairment. Clearance of PER is increased, in patients taking concomitant enzyme inducing AEDs such as phenytoin (PHT) and carbamazepine (CBZ). At a dose of 12 mg, it decreases the efficacy of progesterone-containing hormonal contraception.[4]

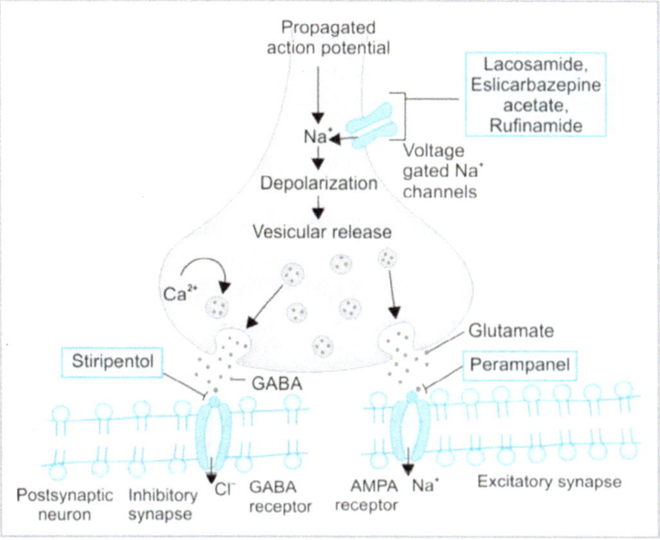

FIG. 1: Lacosamide, eslicarbazepine acetate, rufinamide, steripentol, perampanel mechanism of action.

Dosage and Administration

It is initiated as 2 mg once daily (4 mg with concomitant enzyme inducing AEDs) at bedtime, increasing by 2 mg/day every 1–2 weeks as per tolerance to a maximum dose of 12 mg daily. In geriatric age group, not to exceed beyond 8 mg/day. Pediatric dosage same as adult dosage.

Indication

Perampanel is approved as adjunctive treatment for focal onset seizures with/without secondary generalization in patients aged 4 years and older;[5] and in primary generalized tonic-clonic seizures in patients aged 12 years and older.[6]

Clinical Implications

Perampanel with novel mechanism of action can be useful adjunctive medication for drug resistant epilepsy cases. Once daily dosing is convenient. Cost of therapy is likely to be prohibitive for its use as a first line and even second line agent in most centers.

Side Effects

The most common side effects observed in randomized trials include dizziness, somnolence, headache, fatigue, irritability, nausea and weight gain.[4] Serious dose-dependent neuropsychiatric adverse effects including aggression and hostility may occur. Behavioral and psychiatric side effects have no relation with dose, duration of therapy, rate of titration, concurrent medications, underlying psychiatric and intellectual state.[7] No safety and efficacy data in pregnant and lactating group of patients.

BRIVARACETAM

The mechanism of action of BRV is explained in Figure 2. It is similar to that of levetiracetam (LEV). It binds to the synaptic vesicle protein SV2A, an integral membrane glycoprotein involved in synaptic vesicle exocytosis.[8] BRV has highly selective and reversible affinity for SV2A, occupying 80–90% of SV2A within 5–15 minutes at clinically relevant doses, which represents maximal seizure protection with a 15–30-fold higher affinity for SV2A compared to LEV.[8] Unlike LEV, it does not act on the AMPA and gamma-aminobutyric acid (GABA)-A receptors which is the likely reason for fewer psychiatric side effects.[9] BRV is metabolized in liver to inactive metabolites. BRV may increase the plasma concentrations of PHT and CBZ metabolites via inhibition of epoxide hydroxylase. Conversely, PHT, CBZ, phenobarbital and other CYP2C19 inducers are associated with decreased plasma concentrations of BRV. Dose of BRV needs to be doubled in patients on rifampicin therapy.[10] No interaction with hormonal contraception. In cases with mild-to-moderate liver disease, maximum daily dose not to exceed 150 mg. Not recommended in end-stage renal disease (not studied adequately). Lack of clinical data in terms of safety and efficacy for pregnant and lactating females.

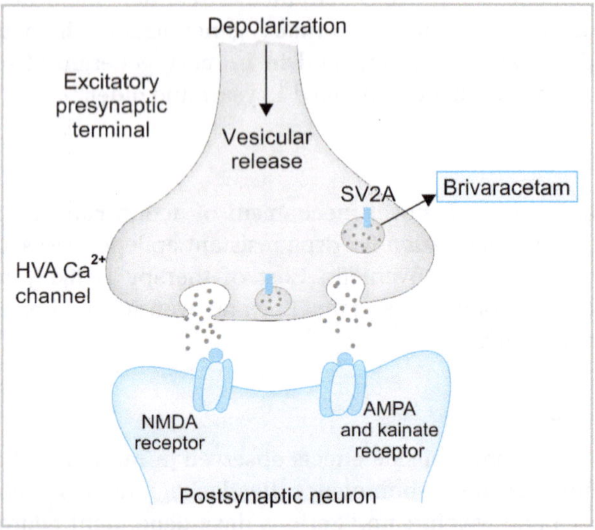

FIG. 2: Brivaracetam mechanism of action.

Dosage and Administration

The drug is available in oral formulations; intravenous formulation is not available in India. The recommended starting dose for adults weighing 50 kg or above is 50 mg twice daily. The dose can be increased to 100 mg twice daily, if needed, based on seizure control. Lower starting dosage recommended in patients with hepatic insufficiency. Pediatric dosage for children weighing 20–49 kg is 4 mg/kg/day PO and for those weighing 11–19 kg is 5 mg/kg/day PO.

Indication

Brivaracetam is approved as monotherapy or adjunctive therapy for focal onset seizures in patients 4 years of age and older.[8] Data suggests BRV is also useful in adults with generalized epilepsy.[11]

Clinical Implications

Brivaracetam has higher efficacy and fewer neuropsychiatric side effects, making it a good alternative to LEV.[12]

Side Effects[13]

The most common side effects are somnolence, dizziness, fatigue and nausea. Psychiatric side effects reported are anxiety, irritability and depression.

LACOSAMIDE

Lacosamide selectively enhances slow inactivation of voltage-gated sodium channels unlike most classic sodium channel blockers, which enhance fast sodium channel.[4] It selectively reduces pathological hyperactivity, while leaving physiological activity intact. LCM targets GABA-A receptors and it can act synergistically with LEV, improve the GABAergic function.[14] This novel mechanism might contribute to explain the clinical efficacy of this combination in several refractory epileptic patients.

Lacosamide has excellent oral bioavailability (~100%) and very low protein binding (15%). LCM is converted in the liver to inactive metabolites, but approximately 40% is eliminated unchanged in the urine. The half-life is approximately 13 hours. LCM is not a significant hepatic-enzyme inducer, but strong cytochrome P450 (CYP) inhibitors (e.g. valproate) may decrease elimination in the presence of hepatic or renal impairment. Dose adjustment should be made in patients with severe hepatic or renal impairment and should be supplemented after hemodialysis. No interactions with hormonal contraceptives.

Lack of clinical data in terms of safety and efficacy for pregnant and lactating females. The mechanism of action of lacosamide is explained in Figure 1.

Indication

Lacosamide is narrow spectrum AED approved as monotherapy and adjunctive therapy for focal onset seizures in adults and children above 4 years of age.[15] Intravenous preparation is being used in status epilepticus.[16]

Clinical Implications

Lacosamide is new drug with a favorable pharmacokinetic profile in terms of safety and absence of any interactions with other majority AEDs or concomitant medications. It is useful in status epilepticus and is being used as second or third line antiepileptic agent.

Dosage and Administration

It is available in oral as well as parenteral formulations. Initiate LCM at a dose of 100 mg/daily in two divided doses. The dose can be titrated as needed by 100 mg every 1–2 weeks to a maintenance dose of 200–400 mg/day. For ages 4–16, start treatment with 1.5 mg/kg twice daily (3 mg/kg/day) for 1 week; increase by 3 mg/kg/day in divided doses as tolerated and as needed at weekly intervals; maximum dose 6 mg/kg twice daily (12 mg/kg/day).

Side Effects

Lacosamide is generally well tolerated. Dizziness, nausea, vertigo, blurred vision, abnormal coordination and ataxia are the most frequently reported side effects. These side effects are compounded when used with other sodium channel blockers like PHT, CBZ and oxcarbazepine (OXC). Dose-dependent PR interval prolongations on electrocardiogram suggest caution in prescribing LCM to those with known conduction problems (e.g. atrioventricular block, sick sinus syndrome) or elderly with concomitant heart problems or on medications that prolong the PR interval.[17]

ESLICARBAZEPINE ACETATE

Eslicarbazepine is a third-generation antiepileptic, structurally similar to CBZ and OXC. Its mechanism of action is explained in Figure 1. It is rapidly converted to the active metabolite S-licarbazepine, the active enantiomer of the OXC. It acts by blocking voltage-gated sodium channels.[18]

It achieves a maximum concentration in 2–3 hours after oral ingestion. Concentrations are unaltered by food. It is not subject to autoinduction. It is metabolized to inactive compounds, but more than 50% is excreted in the urine as unchanged ESL.[4] The half-life of ESL is 13–20 hours. It is a weak inducer of CYP3A4, potentially decreasing plasma concentrations of estrogen and other molecules metabolized by this enzyme, and a weak inhibitor of CYP2C19, potentially increasing plasma concentration of PHT and other drugs metabolized by this enzyme. In turn, PHT or CBZ coadministration reduces level of ESL by enhancing glucoronidation. Warrants increased dosage of oral contraceptives due to enzyme interaction. There is lack of clinical data in terms of efficacy and safety for pregnant and lactating females.

Indication

Eslicarbazepine is approved as monotherapy and adjunctive therapy for focal onset seizures in adults and children as young as 4 years of age.[19]

Clinical Implications

Eslicarbazepine with no pharmacologically active metabolite and once daily dosing is a good alternative monotherapy for focal onset seizures. It has been relaunched in India recently.

Side Effects[20]

Dizziness, drowsiness, nausea, headache, diplopia, ataxia and blurred vision are the most common adverse effects. ESL has been associated with an increase in the PR interval, abnormal liver function tests (LFTs) and hyponatremia.[21] Concomitant treatment with other sodium channel blockers increases the incidence of diplopia, abnormal coordination and dizziness. There are rare incidences of Stevens–Johnson syndrome and toxic epidermal necrolysis and hence ESL should not be used in patients with hypersensitivity to CBZ or PHT.

Dosage and Administration

The recommended starting dose in adults is 400 mg once daily, which can be increased after 1 week to 800 mg daily. The daily dose may be further increased to a maximum of 1,600 mg if warranted and tolerated. Dose adjustment is needed for renal impairment. Its use is not recommended in patients with severe liver impairment. For children above 6 years of age, the recommended starting dose is 10 mg/kg/day once daily.[22] Dosage should be increased in weekly or biweekly increments of 10 mg/kg/day up to 30 mg/kg/day, based on individual response. The maximum dose is 1,200 mg once daily. Children with a body weight of 40 kg or more should be given the same dose as for adults.

RUFINAMIDE

Rufinamide modulates the activity of sodium channels, prolonging the inactive state. Its mechanism of action is explained in Figure 1. This action is particularly effective in depolarized neurons.[23] Pharmacokinetic studies show slow absorption after oral ingestion. Rufinamide is metabolized in liver to pharmacologically inactive metabolites by hydrolysis which is not CYP-dependent. The metabolites are primarily excreted through kidneys. The elimination half-life is 6–10 hours. Enzyme inducing AEDs like CBZ, PHT, primidone (PRM) and phenobarbital may increase the clearance of rufinamide. Valproate is associated with reduced clearance of rufinamide.[24] Rufinamide may reduce the effectiveness of oral hormonal contraceptives.

Dosage and Administration

Adults are treated initially at 400–800 mg/day in two divided doses, increased by 400–800 mg/day every 2 days until maximum daily dose of 3,200 mg is achieved. Lower dosage recommended when patient is on valproic acid. In children, rufinamide is initiated at 10 mg/kg/day in two divided doses, increased by 10 mg/kg increments every other day to a target dose of 45 mg/kg/day.[25]

Indication

Rufinamide is approved by the Food and Drug Administration (FDA) as an adjunctive treatment for seizures associated with Lennox-Gastaut syndrome (LGS).[26] Observational studies suggest rufinamide may have efficacy as an adjunctive therapy in other focal epilepsy and refractory epilepsy syndromes.[27]

Clinical Implications

Rufinamide is an orphan drug approved as an adjunctive therapy for LGS patients. It is too early to ascertain the place of rufinamide in the treatment of other epilepsy syndromes.

Side Effects

The most common side effects are headache, dizziness, fatigue, somnolence, nausea and vomiting. Shortening of the QT interval is seen, hence use should be avoided in patients with congenital short QT syndrome or taking other drugs that shorten the QT interval. Rare hypersensitivity reactions with multi-organ dysfunction have been reported.

STIRIPENTOL

Probably includes potentiation of GABAergic transmission. Its mechanism of action is explained in Figure 1. Precise mechanism behind anticonvulsant effects is unknown. May enhance GABAergic inhibitory neurotransmission by weak partial agonism and/or positive allosteric modulation of GABA-A receptors.[28] Protein binding is almost 99% to plasma proteins. Hepatic metabolism is done through demethylenation, primarily by CYP1A2, 2C19, 3A4 and glucuronidation. Elimination half-life is 4.5–13 hours (dose-dependent); clearance decreases with repeated administration possibly due to inhibition of CYP450 isoenzymes and is markedly decreased at higher doses. Excretion is mainly via kidneys (73% as metabolites); rest via feces (13–24% as unchanged drug).[29] Enzyme-inducing AEDs increase stiripentol clearance by stimulating its metabolism. Stiripentol inhibits the metabolism and increases the serum concentration of phenobarbital, CBZ, PHT, primidone, clobazam (CLB) and valproic acid.[30] As it is usually coprescribed with at least one among valproic acid or CLB in cases of Dravet syndrome (DS), it should be kept in mind.[31]

Dosage and Administration

Maximum oral dosage is 50 mg/kg/day, to be reached over 3 days in two or three divided doses.

Indication

In children and adults with refractory generalized tonic-clonic seizures in DS (severe myoclonic epilepsy in infancy) as add-on with other agents like valproic acid and CLB.[32] No proven efficacy in focal seizures.[33] Some studies indicating better efficacy in DS patients with positive SCN1A mutations.[34]

Clinical Implications

Robust efficacy in DS. Significant drug interactions with complex pharmacokinetics.

Side Effects[35]

Drowsiness, ataxia, tremor, hypotonia, dystonia, hyperactivity, aggressiveness and other behavior disorders, insomnia, nausea, anorexia, weight loss, vomiting and hematological abnormalities (e.g. neutropenia and thrombocytopenia).

CONCLUSION

There is a promising scope for pharmacotherapy in cases of refractory seizures due to the advent of these novel molecules. BRV is an attractive option in cases where behavioral side effects caused by LEV are a major roadblock. In view of the novel mechanism of action of PER, it can be tried in refractory epilepsy cases where there was no seizure control with older molecules. LCM is an upcoming molecule as a rescue agent in intensive care settings in view of availability of intravenous preparations. ESL had added advantage in view of its once a day dosage which can ensure better compliance in patients with chronic epilepsy. Rufinamide and stiripentol are promising agents in cases with refractory seizures in LGS and DS respectively.

REFERENCES

1. Bialer M. New antiepileptic drugs that are second generation to existing antiepileptic drugs. Expert Opin Investig Drugs. 2006;15(6):637-47.
2. Luszczki JJ. Third-generation antiepileptic drugs: mechanisms of action, pharmacokinetics and interactions. Pharmacol Rep. 2009;61(2):197-216.
3. Patsalos PN. The clinical pharmacology profile of the new antiepileptic drug perampanel: A novel noncompetitive AMPA receptor antagonist. Epilepsia. 2015;56(1):12-27 .
4. Patsalos PN, St Louis EK. Epilepsy prescribers guide to antiepileptic drugs, 3rd edition. Cambridge: Cambridge University Press; 2018.
5. De Liso P, Moavero R, Coppola G. et al. Current role of perampanel in pediatric epilepsy. Ital J Pediatr. 2017;43(1):51.
6. French JA, Krauss GL, Wechsler RT, et al. Perampanel for tonic-clonic seizures in idiopathic generalized epilepsy A randomized trial. Neurology. 2015;85(11):950-7.
7. Juhl S, Rubboli G. Add-on perampanel and aggressive behaviour in severe drug-resistant focal epilepsies. Funct Neurol. 2017;32(4):215-20.
8. Stephen LJ, Brodie MJ. Brivaracetam: a novel antiepileptic drug for focal-onset seizures. Ther Adv Neurol Disord. 2017;11:1756285617742081.
9. Klein P, Diaz A, Gasalla T, et al. A review of the pharmacology and clinical efficacy of brivaracetam. Clin Pharmacol. 2018;10:1-22.
10. Stockis A, Watanabe S, Scheen AJ. Effect of rifampin on the disposition of brivaracetam in human subjects: further insights into brivaracetam hydrolysis. Drug Metab Dispos. 2016;44(6):792-9.
11. Grande-Martín A, Sopelana-Garay D, Pardal-Fernández JM, et al. Exceptional response to brivaracetam in a patient with refractory idiopathic generalized epilepsy and absence seizures. Epileptic Disord. 2018;20(1):60-4.
12. Andres E, Kerling F, Hamer H, et al. Behavioural changes in patients with intellectual disability treated with brivaracetam. Acta Neurol Scand.2018;138(3):195-202.
13. Zhu LN, Chen D, Chen T, et al. The adverse event profile of brivaracetam: A meta-analysis of randomized controlled trials. Seizure. 2017;45:7-16.
14. Ruffolo G, Di Bonaventura C, Cifelli P, et al. A novel action of lacosamide on GABAA currents sets the ground for a synergic interaction with levetiracetam in treatment of epilepsy. Neurobiol Dis. 2018;115:59-68.
15. Brigo F. Lacosamide monotherapy for newly diagnosed epilepsy. Lancet Neurol. 2017;16(1):20-2.
16. Husain AM, Lee JW, Kolls BJ, et al. Randomized trial of lacosamide vs fosphenytoin for nonconvulsive seizures. Ann. Neurol. 2018;83(6):1174-85.
17. Bainbridge J, De Backer M, Eckhardt K, et al. Safety and tolerability of lacosamide monotherapy in the elderly: A subgroup analysis from lacosamide trials in diabetic neuropathic pain. Epilepsia Open. 2017;2(4):415-23.
18. Doeser A, Soares-da-Silva P, Beck H, et al. The effects of eslicarbazepine on persistent Na+ current and the role of the Na+ channel β subunits. Epilepsy Res. 2014;108(2):202-11.
19. Lattanzi S, Grillo E, Brigo F, et al. Efficacy and safety of perampanel in Parkinson's disease. A systematic review with meta-analysis. J Neurol. 2018;265(4):733-40.
20. Pazdera L, Sperling MR, Harvey JH, et al. Efficacy and safety of eslicarbazepine acetate monotherapy in patients converting from carbamazepine. Epilepsia. 2018;59(3):704-14.

21. Pulitano P, Franco V, Mecarelli O, et al. Effects of eslicarbazepine acetate on lipid profile and sodium levels in patients with epilepsy. Seizure. 2017;53:1-3.
22. Lattanzi S, Brigo F, Cagnetti C, et al. Eslicarbazepine acetate in the treatment of adults with partial-onset epilepsy: an evidence-based review of efficacy, safety and place in therapy. Core Evid. 2018;13:21-31.
23. Panebianco M, Prabhakar H, Marson AG. Rufinamide add-on therapy for refractory epilepsy. Cochrane Database Syst Rev. 2018;4:CD011772.
24. Arzimanoglou, A. et al. Safety and pharmacokinetic profile of rufinamide in pediatric patients aged less than 4 years with Lennox-Gastaut syndrome: An interim analysis from a multicenter, randomized, active-controlled, open-label study. Eur J Paediatr Neurol. 2016;20(3):393-402.
25. Kothare S, Kluger G, Sachdeo R, et al. Dosing considerations for rufinamide in patients with Lennox-Gastaut syndrome: Phase III trial results and real-world clinical data. Seizure. 2017;47:25-33.
26. Coppola G, Besag F, Cusmai R, et al. Current role of rufinamide in the treatment of childhood epilepsy: literature review and treatment guidelines. Eur J Paediatr Neurol. 2014;18(6):685-90.
27. Jaraba S, Santamarina E, Miró J, et al. Rufinamide in children and adults in routine clinical practice. Acta Neurol Scand. 2017;135(1):122-8.
28. Stiripentol (Diacomit): For Severe Myoclonic Epilepsy in Infancy (Dravet Syndrome). Ottawa (ON): Canadian Agency for Drugs and Technologies in Health, 2015.
29. Shorvon S, Perucca E, Engel Jr J (Eds). The Treatment of Epilepsy, 4th edition. Hoboken: Wiley; 2015.
30. Verrotti A, Prezioso G, Stagi S, et al. Pharmacological considerations in the use of stiripentol for the treatment of epilepsy. Expert Opin Drug Metab Toxicol. 2016;12(3):345-52.
31. Jogamoto T, Yamamoto Y, Fukuda M, et al. Add-on stiripentol elevates serum valproate levels in patients with or without concomitant topiramate therapy. Epilepsy Res. 2017;130:7-12.
32. Nickels KC, Wirrell EC. Stiripentol in the management of epilepsy. CNS Drugs. 2017;31(5):405-16.
33. Brigo F, Igwe SC, Bragazzi NL. Stiripentol add-on therapy for focal refractory epilepsy. Cochrane Database Syst Rev. 2018;5:CD009887.
34. Cho MJ, Kwon SS, Ko A, et al. Efficacy of Stiripentol in Dravet Syndrome with or without SCN1A Mutations. J Clin Neurol. 2018;14(1):22-8.
35. Myers KA, Lightfoot P, Patil SG, et al. Stiripentol efficacy and safety in Dravet syndrome: a 12-year observational study. Dev Med Child Neurol. 2018;60(6):574-8.

6

CHAPTER

Antiepileptic Drug Therapy in Children

Yeeshu S Sudan, Atma Ram Bansal

INTRODUCTION

Epilepsy in pediatric age group is diverse with different etiologies. As far as treatment is concerned, role of antiepileptic drugs (AEDs) is same as in adult age group. However, due to different causes and pharmacokinetics in pediatric age group, some drugs are used more frequently than others. At the same time, many AEDs have their special role in specific age group among children. Modern day's AEDs have recently gained momentum in pediatric age group due to better adverse reaction profile and lesser drug interactions.

Since accurate identification is the key to successful treatment, it is proposed that pediatric epilepsy can be divided into three etiological and prognostic groups. Early identification of these groups can help in managing various pediatric epileptic disorders. This also helps in prognostication of disorder and counseling the parents in better way. These groups are benign epilepsies of childhood, pharmacodependent epilepsies and pharmacoresistant epilepsies. The special group of neonatal seizures is also discussed in detail. The chapter also discusses management guidelines on West syndrome.

BENIGN EPILEPSIES OF CHILDHOOD

These constitute idiopathic, benign syndromes and affect almost one-fourth of pediatric epilepsy population with nonfebrile seizures. This group includes:

- Benign childhood epilepsy with centrotemporal spikes (BCECTSs) or rolandic epilepsy
- Early-onset benign childhood occipital epilepsy (Panayiotopoulos type)
- Late-onset childhood occipital epilepsy (Gastaut type)
- Childhood absence epilepsy
- Benign childhood seizure susceptibility syndrome.

These patients present with nocturnal seizures which may be missed initially. Their neurological development is normal but few may have positive family history of epilepsy or febrile seizures. Electroencephalogram (EEG) is grossly abnormal in these patients and epileptiform discharges may be seen especially during sleep record. However, if clinical seizures are not frequent (or mild and nocturnal), treatment is usually not required. Since these are age-limited disorders, if seizure onset is close to the natural age of remission of this, long-term treatment with AEDs can be avoided. Treatment is required only in those with frequent seizures, secondarily generalized tonic-clonic seizures (GTCSs) or comorbid conditions. Carbamazepine and sodium valproate are found to be effective and is considered as drug of choice in these conditions. Some patients (mainly atypical benign rolandic epilepsy) can have paradoxical response to carbamazepine and hence a repeat EEG and change of AED is required if there is clinical worsening. Levetiracetam is emerging as a good alternative in this condition. If seizures are refractory, other drugs for focal epilepsies can be considered. It is important to note that EEG may remain abnormal for many years after the onset of epilepsy even when child is seizure-free. Hence repeating EEG once seizures are controlled leads to confusion and overtreatment; and it should be avoided.

Most children suffering from benign focal epilepsy have an excellent prognosis. Up to 80–90% of patients may have only single or very infrequent seizures. Only 10–20% of patients may have frequent seizures, which may be refractory to treatment. Remission of benign childhood focal seizures is expected by the age of 15–16 years.

Childhood Absence Epilepsy

Typical absence epilepsy is seen in otherwise normal children of between 4 and 8 years and is genetically determined. Usually these absences are very frequent occurring multiple times per day. EEG hallmarks of absences are symmetrical, synchronous and bilateral 3 Hz spike-wave discharges which are triggered during hyperventilation against a normal background. Most patients in this respond to single drug (or occasionally two drugs) in appropriate dose. Valproate or ethosuximide as monotherapy are the drugs of choice and effective in majority of the children. In case of failure or resistance to these drugs, lamotrigine, levetiracetam and zonisamide are the reasonable alternatives. Combination of lamotrigine and valproate is effective in resistant cases. Drugs like carbamazepine, gabapentin, oxcarbazepine, phenytoin, phenobarbital, pregabalin, tiagabine and vigabatrin can aggravate seizures and should be avoided. Spontaneous remission is seen after a few years.

PHARMACODEPENDENT EPILEPSIES

This group of idiopathic generalized epilepsy (IGE) constitutes 20% of pediatric epilepsy population. Drug treatment controls the seizures in this group of patients but there is no spontaneous remission. Common examples are:

- Juvenile myoclonic epilepsy (JME)
- Juvenile absence epilepsy
- Epilepsy with myoclonic absences
- Epilepsy with GTCS only.

Recurrence of seizures on stopping or reducing the dose of drug is the characteristic feature of all these epilepsies. Occasionally instead of monotherapy, combination of synergistic drugs is required to control seizures in these patients. Wrong diagnosis is very common in this group of disorder which leads to administration of inappropriate AED. This results in intractability and morbidity (and even mortality). Focal onset seizures with secondary generalization should be excluded after proper history and EEG.

Many AEDs licensed for focal epilepsies are initiated in IGE which leads to exacerbation of seizures. Sometimes, a particular drug is effective in seizure type and worsens other seizure type in same patient. Therefore, in case of multiple seizure type, it is imperative to understand which seizure type predominates. For example, if carbamazepine, oxcarbazepine or phenytoin are used in IGE, this may result in exacerbation of absences and myoclonic jerks. Clonazepam effectively controls myoclonic jerks, but is not effective in primary GTCSs. On the other hand, lamotrigine may exacerbate myoclonic jerk but effectively controls primary GTCSs. Valproate and levetiracetam are probably the two drugs which have shown no specific contraindication in any group. Second-generation drugs like topiramate and zonisamide are also used increasingly and effectively in patients with multiple seizure types. The third-generation drugs are not yet used frequently because of lack of literature evidence. Nevertheless, it would be exciting to see how these drugs would fit themselves in spectrum of these disorders.

PHARMACORESISTANT EPILEPSIES

This group constitutes an important part of epilepsy management. Epilepsies in this group are quite heterogeneous in terms of etiological diagnosis and prognosis. Between 15% and 20% all epilepsy patients fall under this category. The two major subsets are:

1. Epileptic encephalopathies
2. Focal symptomatic epilepsy.

Epileptic encephalopathies are often resistant to treatment and many a times considered as catastrophic epilepsies. In these cases, seizures are often polymorphic and intractable along with significant cognitive, behavioral and neurological deficits. Seizure may be seen even from first day of life. These disorders are age specific and present during a particular age period. Early myoclonic encephalopathy and Ohtahara syndrome present during neonatal and early infancy age group. Similarly, West syndrome presents typically during 4–6 months of life. On the other hand, Dravet syndrome, Doose syndrome and Lennox-Gastaut syndrome (LGS) present after first year of life and contribute of substantial morbidity during early childhood.

Epileptic encephalopathies with continuous spike-and-wave during sleep (CSWS) including Landau-Kleffner syndrome (LKS) are rare epileptic encephalopathy syndromes which are seen in early childhood as predominant behavior change rather than frequent seizures.

Other known syndromes which are pharmacoresistant include Rasmussen's syndrome, migrating partial epilepsy of early childhood, hemiconvulsion-hemiplegia, gelastic seizures with hypothalamic hamartoma. Likewise, genetic epilepsy like *CDKL5, PCDH19* mutation in ion channel genes (sodium, calcium, potassium) and plethora of recently detected genes represent subgroup which may be resistant to drug treatment.

ANTIEPILEPTIC DRUGS

The history, type of seizure and EEG findings help in identifying the right kind of drug. Use of single drug with minimal side effects and complete control of seizures should be the ultimate treatment goal. The main principal of treatment is to start low and go slow, i.e. to start with lowest possible dose and escalate the dose slowly until seizures are controlled or side effects develop.

There is a long list of first-generation AEDs available for the treatment of epilepsy in children. Available first-generation drugs are carbamazepine, valproic acid, phenytoin, phenobarbital, clobazam, clonazepam and ethosuximide. Of second-generation AEDs, levetiracetam, oxcarbazepine, lamotrigine, topiramate, felbamate, tiagabine, vigabatrin, zonisamide, etc. are approved by the Food and Drug Administration (FDA). The most recently approved third-generation newer drugs are lacosamide, eslicarbazepine acetate, rufinamide, stiripentol, perampanel, etc. Table 1 depicts the doses, mechanism of action, indications and side effect profile of commonly used AEDs.

TABLE 1: Doses, mechanism of action, indications and side effect profile of commonly used antiepileptic drugs.

Drug	Loading dose or starting dose	Maintenance dose	Mechanism of action	Clinical use	Common side effects
Phenobarbitone	10–20 mg/kg/day in two divided doses (IV or oral)	3–8 mg/kg/day once or twice daily	Dec Na^+, dec Ca^{2+}, inc GABA, dec glutamate	Broad spectrum	Drowsiness, sedation, impairment of cognition and hyperkinetic behavior, rash, hepatic failure
Phenytoin	10–20 mg/kg/day in two divided doses (IV or oral)	5–10 mg/kg/day twice daily	Blocking voltage-dependent Na^+ channels	Broad spectrum	Ataxia, drowsiness, lethargy, sedation, gingival hyperplasia, hirsutism, rickets, osteomalacia, rash
Valproic acid	10 mg/kg/day in two divided doses (IV or oral)	10–40 mg/kg/day twice daily	Dec Na^+, dec Ca^{2+}, inc GABA, dec glutamate	Broad spectrum (GTCS >Focal)	Nausea, vomiting, weight gain, tremor, hair loss, hepatic and pancreatic failure
Carbamazepine	8–10 mg/kg/day twice or thrice daily	20–40 mg/kg/day twice or thrice daily	Blocking voltage-dependent Na^+ channels	Focal epilepsies	Rash, sedation, ataxia, nystagmus, tremor, hyponatremia, cardiac arrhythmia, hematological
Oxcarbazepine	8–10 mg/kg/day twice or thrice daily	20–40 mg/kg/day twice or thrice daily	Blocking voltage-dependent Na^+ channels	Focal epilepsies	Rash, sedation, ataxia, nystagmus, tremor, hyponatremia, cardiac arrhythmia
Levetiracetam	10–20 mg/kg/day twice or thrice daily	20–60 mg/kg/day twice or thrice daily	Binding to synaptic vesicle protein SV2A	Broad spectrum	Behavioral and psychotic changes, irritability, dizziness, somnolence
Clobazam	0.1–0.3 mg/kg/day once or twice daily	0.1–1 mg/kg/day once or twice daily	Inc GABA	Broad spectrum (Focal >GTCS)	Sedation, drowsiness, cognitive impairment, aggressiveness, hypersalivation, coordination disturbances, tolerance and withdrawal syndrome
Clonazepam	0.01–0.02 mg/kg/day once or twice daily	0.1–0.2 mg/kg/day once or twice daily	Inc GABA	Broad spectrum (Focal >GTCS)	Sedation, drowsiness, cognitive impairment, aggressiveness, hypersalivation, coordination disturbances, tolerance and withdrawal syndrome

(Continued)

(Continued)

Drug	Loading dose or starting dose	Maintenance dose	Mechanism of action	Clinical use	Common side effects
Topiramate	0.5–1 mg/kg/day once or twice daily	1–5 mg/kg/day once or twice daily	Dec Na^+, dec Ca^{2+}	Focal and secondary generalized	Anhidrosis, anorexia, fatigue, nervousness, difficulty with concentration/attention, memory impairment, metabolic acidosis, weight loss, renal calculi, acute angle-closure glaucoma
Zonisamide	1–2 mg/kg/day	4–12 mg/kg/day	Dec Na^+, dec Ca^{2+}	Focal and secondary generalized	Anhidrosis, drowsiness, anorexia, irritability, weight loss, renal calculi
Vigabatrin	25–50 mg/kg/day twice daily	50–200 mg/kg/day twice daily	Irreversible GABA transaminase inhibitor	Infantile spasms, tuberous sclerosis	Irreversible visual field defects, fatigue, weight gain
Ethosuximide	5–10 mg/kg/day twice or thrice daily	20–35 mg/kg/day twice or thrice daily	Blocking T-type Ca^{2+} channels	Absence epilepsy	Gastrointestinal disturbances, anorexia, weight loss, drowsiness
Lamotrigine	0.2 mg/kg/day once or twice daily	1–5 mg/kg given (slow increment in doses)		Broad spectrum (Focal >GTCS)	Life-threatening rash, tics, insomnia, dizziness, diplopia, headache, ataxia, asthenia
Stiripentol	10 mg/kg/day	10–50 mg/kg/day	Inc GABA levels	Dravet syndrome	Anorexia, weight loss, insomnia, drowsiness, ataxia, hypotonia, dystonia
Rufinamide	10 mg/kg/day twice daily	45 mg/kg/day twice daily	Prolong the inactive state of Na^+	Lennox-Gastaut syndrome, epileptic encephalopathies	Headache, dizziness, fatigue, ataxia

(Dec: decrease; Inc: increase; IV: intravenous; Na^+: sodium channel; Ca^{2+}: calcium channel; GABA: gamma-aminobutyric acid; GTCS: generalized tonic-clonic seizure)

Because of lack of evidence concerning safety and efficacy, role of second- and third-generation AEDs is limited to off-label second-line option in pediatric population. Unfortunately, for children younger than 2 years of age, the studies are very limited. Though this group of children also suffer from refractory seizures associated with severe epileptic encephalopathies of varied genetic etiologies, there are not many guidelines on use of various AEDs in this population.

Among the first-line AEDs, valproic acid, carbamazepine, phenytoin and phenobarbitone are the commonly used drugs for variety of epileptic conditions. Since valproic acid has shown broad-spectrum efficacy, it can be used in all childhood epilepsies either focal or generalized, but is a preferred choice in GTCSs. For focal seizures, carbamazepine is still considered a first-line drug; however, newer drugs are increasing used as first line in this group. It should be noted that carbamazepine could worsen seizures when used in certain generalized or unclassifiable epilepsies like absence or myoclonic epilepsy.[1]

Clobazam is reserved for use in refractory focal epilepsies. It is found to be effective in reducing atonic seizures and total seizure frequency in LGS and other complex epilepsies. It has been gradually more and more used as an add-on drug in refractory group.

Since there are no significant side effects and drug-drug interaction, levetiracetam is being frequently drug nowadays. It can be used as first line or add-on to other AEDs to treat focal seizures with or without generalization in patients more than 1 month of age. It is also one of the drugs of choice for JME and IGE in patients 12 years and above. While topiramate is considered as a good option for monotherapy or add-on therapy in patients above 2 years of age with focal seizures or GTCS, its use in routine clinical practice is limited because of many side effects like concentration difficulties, speech issues, weight loss, ataxia and paresthesias.

Vigabatrin is approved as monotherapy in the treatment of infantile spasms since 2009. It is considered to be superior to hydrocortisone and is first-line choice when spasms are seen in patients suffering from tuberous sclerosis.[2] However, negative impact on visual field needs to be monitored regularly. Zonisamide is extensively used clinically as it has broad-spectrum properties. Besides primary GTCS, it is effective in focal seizures with or without GTCSs and epileptic spasms of West syndrome. Loss of sweating, formation of renal calculus, loss of appetite and weight, and cognitive impairment are the major side effects.

Of recently approved drugs, perampanel[3] is being used as add-on therapy to treat primary generalized epilepsy as well as focal seizure with or without secondary generalization in patients above 12 years of age. Dizziness, ataxia, falls, and depressive symptoms like irritability, suicidal tendencies, fatigue, drowsiness, etc. are the major side effects. Rufinamide[4] is another drug approved as add-on therapy in children above 4 years of age with refractory focal epilepsy and in LGS.[3] Similarly, Stiripentol is used in severe myoclonic epilepsy of infancy (SMEI or Dravet syndrome) as an adjunctive to clobazam and valproic acid to treat refractory GTCS. However, long-term efficacy and tolerability of this drug is not yet known.

Finally, cannabidiol (CBD), the nonpsychotropic compound of *Cannabis sativa* is found to have anticonvulsant properties and appears to be safe in anecdotal reports. However, legal restrictions and nonavailability of pure, pharmacologically active compounds have restricted its use in clinical practice.[5]

NEONATAL AGE GROUP

Seizures are more common in the neonatal period because brain is immature and can badly affect neurodevelopmental outcome. Recurrent seizures predispose the child to cognitive and behavioral complications in later life.

Symptomatic causes like hypoglycemia, hypocalcemia and hypomagnesemia are responsible for majority of the cases and require specific treatment of the underlying cause rather than AEDs. Similarly, there are certain seizure mimickers in this age group which do not require any treatment (benign sleep myoclonus and neonatal tremors). Unnecessary treatment should be avoided in these conditions. Clinical semiology to define the seizure types along with EEG monitoring is necessary to determine underlying topography which may help in deciding when not to treat.

On the other hand, disorders like meningitis, encephalitis or structural causes such as hypoxic-ischemic encephalopathy (HIE) and malformation of brain can lead to recurrent seizures and require antiseizure medications.

While older AEDs like phenobarbitone, phenytoin and benzodiazepines are still commonly used by pediatricians, there is increase surge in use of newer AEDs in this age group recently. Because of better safety profile and few drug interactions, levetiracetam and/or topiramate are the frequently used newer AEDs in neonates.[6]

Phenytoin should be avoided in newborn with hypotension and those who are on vasopressors because it has got potential to cause myocardial depression. Phenobarbitone, on the other hand, increases the electroclinical dissociation; though clinical seizures may decrease, a number of electrographic seizures increase after its use.[7] While lidocaine is more effective compared to benzodiazepines in controlling status epilepticus, it has narrow therapeutic window. Hence it can cause cardiac arrhythmias or hypotension; and paradoxically it can even induce seizures at high doses.[8]

A therapeutic trial with pyridoxine, pyridoxal 5'-phosphate, and folinic acid is mandated in all cases with recurrent seizures or persistent EEG background abnormalities,[9] especially in case of normal magnetic resonance imaging (MRI) of the brain and metabolic profile.

MANAGEMENT OF WEST SYNDROME AND TUBEROUS SCLEROSIS COMPLEX

Once the diagnosis of West syndrome is confirmed on EEG, it is imperative to start the treatment as early as possible. Total control of the clinical events as well as disappearance of hypsarrhythmia or modified hypsarrhythmia on video EEG are two major goals of therapy.

The etiological diagnosis is important because it would help to strategize management option, guide therapeutic decisions and help provide a more definitive prognosis for the child. Usually HIE is a common cause scenario in developing countries. However, other causes such as tuberous sclerosis, chromosomal, stroke, malformation of cortical development, antenatal and perinatal infections also contribute significant numbers. Treatment is also directed by the etiology of the spasms. Vigabatrin is superior to steroids in controlling seizures in patients with tuberous sclerosis complex (TSC). Even in patients without TSC, combining steroids to vigabatrin seems to be more effective in stopping epileptic spasms than hormonal therapy alone. Hence all patients without known TSC should be offered combination therapy with vigabatrin and steroids while patients with known TSC should be offered vigabatrin monotherapy as first line.

Prednisolone should be given in dose of 10 mg four times a day for 14 days. If spasms continue on day 7, or reappear between day 7 and day 14, the dose should be increased to 20 mg three times a day for the remaining days. Steroid weaning should start on day 15, regardless of whether spasms continue or abnormal EEG persists. Tapering should be done on weekly basis over several weeks with 10 mg reduction every week. On the other hand, vigabatrin is given orally, twice a day starting with 50 mg/kg/day increasing every 2–3 days at an incremental dose of 25–50 mg/kg/day to reach a maximum of 150–200 mg/kg/day. If effective, vigabatrin dose will remain same for 3 months. If child has responded to the initial treatment by day 14, vigabatrin weaning can be started after 3 months from initiation of treatment. At 3 months, wean vigabatrin over 4–6 weeks. Major side effect of vigabatrin is concentric constriction of visual field which is bilateral, affecting nasal half more than temporal one. It is seen in 30–40% of cases receiving it for 6 months or more. Ophthalmologic assessment with electroretinogram should be sought for cases on prolonged therapy.

If the child is not responding to steroids and vigabatrin, second line of medication should be tried. Cofactor deficiency such as pyridoxine, pyridoxal 5'-phosphate, folinic acid, should be kept in mind in unresponsive cases and is worth trying.

Other medication which may have some role includes sodium valproate, topiramate, zonisamide, clobazam and ketogenic diet (KD). Epilepsy surgery has important role to play in cases of structural malformation and in cases of tuberous sclerosis where early surgery may give dramatic results in controlling seizures and give child a chance for normal development.

ROLE OF OTHER THERAPIES

Antiepileptic drugs do not fully control seizures, hence cannot change the outcome in most cases. Early treatment sometimes may offer hope to control seizure and make way for normal development. Sometimes, only seizure control is not the aim; as abnormal EEG may contribute to regression or stagnation of development, repeat EEG and close surveillance is required in all such cases.

Despite, treating aggressively with drugs, most of the epileptic encephalopathy children are left with significant comorbidity in terms of cognitive, motor and behavior skills.

Polytherapy is often required usually in higher doses with notable side effects. In many instances, seizure reduction rather than seizure control is the aim to keep the child out of drug-induced behavioral issues. Another point to be noted is that drug-induced worsening is common with polymorphic seizures. Therefore, it is important to know which seizure type is predominant and which type of AED will be most effective for that particular type.

Epilepsy surgery is gaining momentum due to its ability to cure the disease, especially if lesion is evident on MRI. For instance, focal cortical dysplasia and tuberous sclerosis lesions are surgically amenable in most cases. Moreover, palliative surgical and nonsurgical options (vagal nerve stimulation, deep brain stimulation and responsive neurostimulation) have shown some hope in seizure reduction and better social life; hence are gaining popularity. Nonepileptic medications such as steroids, adrenocorticotropic hormone (ACTH), intravenous immunoglobulin may play role in controlling seizures in West syndrome, resistant cases of LGS, CSWS, LKS and occasionally, in patients with status epilepticus. Nonpharmacological treatment options such as KD are being used more frequently in epilepsy clinics. In KD, fat is the major source of energy, while carbohydrate content is very low but protein content is adequate. Few cases of Dravet syndrome, myoclonic-atonic epilepsy and glucose transporter type 1 (GLUT1) deficiency syndrome have shown dramatic results and patients became seizures free with KD.

REFERENCES

1. National Institute for Health and Care Excellence. (2012). The epilepsies: the diagnosis and management of the epilepsies in adults and children in primary and secondary care. [online] Available from: http://www.nice.org.uk/guidance/cg137
2. Chiron C, Dumas C, Jambaque I, et al. Randomized trial comparing vigabatrin and hydrocortisone in infantile spasms due to tuberous sclerosis. Epilepsy Res. 1997;26:389-95.
3. Biton V, Krauss G, Vasquez-Santana B, et al. A randomized, double-blind, placebo-controlled, parallel-group study of rufinamide as adjunctive therapy for refractory partial-onset seizures. Epilepsia. 2011;52:234-42.
4. Kramer LD, Satlin A, Krauss GL, et al. Perampanel for adjunctive treatment of partial-onset seizures: a pooled dose-response analysis of phase III studies. Epilepsia. 2014;55:423-31.
5. Cilio MR, Thiele EA, Devinsky O. The case for assessing cannabidiol in epilepsy. Epilepsia. 2014;55(6):787-90.
6. Silverstein FS, Ferriero DM. Off-label use of antiepileptic drugs for the treatment of neonatal seizures. Pediatr Neurol. 2008;39:77-9.
7. Scher M, Alvin J, Gaus L, et al. Uncoupling of EEG-clinical neonatal seizures after antiepileptic drug use. Pediatr Neurol. 2003;28:277-80.
8. Van Rooij LG, Toet MC, Rademaker KM, et al. Cardiac arrhythmias in neonates receiving lidocaine as anticonvulsive treatment. Eur J Pediatr. 2004;163:637-41.
9. Rosati A, De Masi S, Guerrini R. Antiepileptic drug treatment in children with epilepsy. CNS Drugs. 2015;29:847-63.

7

CHAPTER

Antiepileptic Drugs in Geriatric Population

Vivek Mathew

INTRODUCTION

Elderly patients with epilepsy are more likely to have comorbidities and be on other medications besides having age related alteration of pharmacodynamics. This makes prescribing antiepileptic drugs (AEDs) a greater challenge, requiring us to know all possible metabolic abnormalities and comorbidities in a given patient as well as the relevant pharmacology of each AED. Ultimately, efficacy and safety must be balanced and individualized.

DEFINITION OF ELDERLY

Our use of chronological age of 65 years for "elderly" is arbitrary. When discussing pharmacotherapy, we are more interested in the physiological changes of aging. The Western definitions are often based on urban retirement age concept, or the age at which the population becomes eligible for various financial benefits or concessions.

BURDEN OF EPILEPSY IN ELDERLY

Nearly 25% of new onset seizures occur in individuals over the age of 65 years.[1,2] A cohort was followed up in Rochester, Minnesota from 1935 onwards. On analysis till 1967, it was found that the incidence of new cases of epilepsy in adults remained almost constant at around 15 per 100,000 till the age of 60 years, but rose to 50 after age of 60 years and to 75 per 100,000 population beyond 70 years.[3] In North American and European registries, the incidence of epilepsy in elderly ranged from 1 to 3 per 1,000 person-years[4-7] and prevalence of epilepsy from 2 to 5%.[8,9]

The clinical manifestations and etiology of seizures and epilepsy differ in elderly and influence the diagnostic and therapeutic approach. Elderly are more susceptible to adverse effects of AEDs and are more likely to have multiple medical comorbidities and to be on multiple medications. Quality of life implications also differ in older patients, being vulnerable to loss of independence, and risk of falls. At time of new-onset seizures, they may be living independently or in a nursing home or admitted in a hospital for treatment of other illnesses. This makes the prescription of AEDs for elderly challenging.

HOW IS THE APPROACH TO TREATMENT OF EPILEPSY DIFFERENT IN ELDERLY POPULATION?

Causes and Diagnosis

Diseases of the elderly predispose them to both acute symptomatic seizures and epilepsy. About half (50%) of the acute symptomatic seizures in elderly are related to stroke. Metabolic encephalopathies (6–30%), drugs including drug withdrawal (10%) are the next most common causes.[10-12]

Stroke is also the most common cause for epilepsy in the elderly. It is a known cause in 30–50% of patients and thought to be the underlying factor even in those where the cause is not clearly known.[1,5,7,10,12-14] Alzheimer's disease is associated with increased risk of seizures, ten times higher than expected for same age group.[15-17]

The most important differentials for seizures in the elderly are syncope, transient ischemic attacks (TIAs, including limb shaking TIAs), transient global amnesia (TGA), drop attacks, psychogenic, delirium and rapid eye movement (REM) sleep behavioral disorders.[18-24]

Type of Seizure

The most common type of seizure is focal followed by bilateral tonic clonic.[25] Idiopathic generalized epilepsy with onset in elderly is described but not as common.[26] Focal seizure with impaired awareness was the most common seizure type in a Veteran Affairs Hospital study.[27] Focal seizures with impaired awareness are more often extratemporal and thus with atypical manifestations,[28] and postictal states are often prolonged.[29]

Age-related Pharmacokinetics

Elderly have reduced gastric acid secretion, increase in gastric emptying and intestinal transit time, reduced mesenteric flow and intestinal absorptive surface area.[30] The frequent use of antacids in the elderly further impairs absorption of several AEDs especially phenytoin.[31] There are concerns about absorption of some of the newer anticonvulsants, particularly gabapentin due to its using a saturable amino acid transporter system.[32]

TABLE 1: Antiepileptic drugs metabolized by hepatic enzyme systems.

Primarily P450	Partial P450	Glucuronidation
Carbamazepine, oxcarbazepine, phenobarbital, phenytoin, zonisamide	Topiramate, valproate	Valproate, lamotrigine, active metabolite of oxcarbazepine

Albumin levels can be reduced in sick elderly and with suboptimal nutrition. The free fraction of highly protein-bound AED will increase with increase in adverse effects without proportionate change in total serum level. This is true for phenytoin, valproate, diazepam, clonazepam, clobazam and to a lesser extent, carbamazepine.[33]

The hepatic cytochrome P450 system declines in efficiency with age in an unpredictable manner. The drugs metabolized *primarily* by this system include carbamazepine, oxcarbazepine, phenytoin, phenobarbital and zonisamide. Topiramate and valproate also utilize this system. The hepatic glucuronidation conjugation system declines much less with age, and the AEDs *primarily* undergoing conjugation are lamotrigine and valproate (Table 1).[34]

Decline in renal clearance is, among the most consistent of age-related changes, influencing pharmacokinetics. The AEDs that are *primarily* renally excreted include levetiracetam, gabapentin and pregabalin. Zonisamide and topiramate are *partially* renally excreted.[34]

Comorbid Conditions, Comedications and Drug Interactions

The Iowa 65+ Rural Health Study found nearly 90% of elderly patients in the community taking at least one prescription medicine.[35] Nursing home residents were taking an average of five medications.[31] The major drug interactions are based upon the cytochrome P450 enzyme inducing or inhibiting effects of the AEDs. A simplified table is presented in the chapter (Table 2). In general, levetiracetam, gabapentin, pregabalin, zonisamide, lamotrigine and topiramate have lower potential for drug interactions.[36]

On the other hand, rifampicin is an example of a potent hepatic enzyme *inducer* and can lead to loss of efficacy of many AEDs that are dependent on the hepatic enzyme system for their own metabolism. Commonly used *inhibitors* of the cytochrome P450 system include H2 blockers, macrolide antibiotics, antifungal agents and isoniazid. These can raise the levels of hepatic metabolized AEDs to toxic levels.[36]

TABLE 2: Effects of antiepileptic drugs on hepatic enzyme systems (simplified).

Potent inducers	Mild inducers	Potent inhibitor	Neither inducer nor inhibitor
Phenobarbital, phenytoin, carbamazepine	Felbamate, oxcarbazepine, topiramate	Valproate	Ethosuximide, gabapentin, lamotrigine, levetiracetam, zonisamide, pregabalin

Impact of Seizures and AED on Elderly

Having a seizure or the possibility of having a second seizure in the elderly can have its own physical and psychological consequences. The potential for disability is contributed by the risk of falls, poorer bone health, and increased risk for fractures related to the seizure per se. Falls can be due to both seizures and medication effects. The Osteoporotic Fractures Research Group studied 8,000 elderly women in the community and found that those taking AEDs were 75% more likely to experience a fall than others.[37] This increase can only partly be attributed to seizures, as the AED can contribute to imbalance and falls.

The fracture risk in patients with epilepsy is double that of general population.[38] The bone mineral density (BMD) also declines significantly with AEDs that are potent inducers of the hepatic P450 enzyme system. This includes phenytoin, carbamazepine and phenobarbital.[39] Thus, it could be hypothesized that valproate which is an inhibitor of this enzyme system should be protective for bone health. However, this was not borne out by studies of BMD at metacarpal, which found valproate-related loss of bone mineral was comparable to phenytoin.[40]

The effect of lamotrigine on bone health is not clear. While elevated osteocalcin (marker for bone formation) has been found in patients on lamotrigine, there was no reduction in BMD.[41,42] Data is limited on effect of zonisamide, topiramate and levetiracetam on bone health.[43]

The relationship of seizures in elderly and cognitive decline has also been studied. Age-accelerated memory impairment has been found in patients with chronic intractable temporal lobe epilepsy who have the apoE-e4 allele.[44] Dementias including Alzheimer's have been shown to be significantly associated with epilepsy in some population-based studies.[45,46]

Treatment Outcomes in Elderly

Studies on prognosis of epilepsy in elderly have not been consistent. A Scandinavian study reported 72% of new onset seizures in elderly going into remission within the 1st year.[47] The Veterans Affairs study found seizure free rates of around 50%, which was not different from general population.[27] The UK Lamotrigine Elderly Study Group found only 33% seizure free in the final 16 weeks, probably contributed by higher rates of medication withdrawal, suggesting seizures are not so easy to control.[48]

ALGORITHMS

Whether to Start AED (or Stop AED) or not?

The diagnosis of a seizure in the elderly is made difficult by the variety of potential mimics and the often atypical manifestations of seizures. When we consider the potential for harm by medicines, the decision to start AED becomes difficult.

The questions to be answered when dealing with a possible seizure in the older patient are not different from any other age. The way the questions are answered may be different.

1. *How certain are we that this was a seizure and not a mimic?* Syncope in elderly can be associated with less typical features including prolonged postictal recovery and ictal clonic jerks. History may not be reliable in elderly staying alone. There are multiple potential causes for syncope in the elderly. This includes postural hypotension due to drugs, cardiac arrhythmias and carotid sinus sensitivity.[49] Urinary incontinence during the event is not uncommon in syncope. While there are many clinical pointers toward syncope versus seizure, the most specific would be to capture an event either during prolonged video electroencephalography (EEG) monitoring or head-up tilt table test.

   Transient global amnesia is a clinical syndrome characterized by a memory loss without other cognitive dysfunction for a variable duration of a few minutes to hours. The underlying pathophysiology is likely heterogenous, and includes vascular, migraine related and epileptic phenomena as possible mechanisms.[50] MRI findings of punctate diffusion restricting signal changes in hippocampi may not be specific.[51]

   Focal seizures causing transient global amnesia are more likely to be associated with impaired awareness, but this can be difficult to determine. Prolonged EEG monitoring can help in those with recurrent TGA. An entity called "epileptic pseudodementia" has been described, which is focal seizure with impaired awareness masquerading as dementia.[52] History of 1–25 years duration of fluctuating memory loss and confusion has been described. Prolonged EEG monitoring is needed to pick up the electrographic seizures.

Psychogenic nonepileptic events have been described in elderly as well. In a cohort of 94 patients over the age of 60 years referred for video EEG for paroxysmal events, 27 had nonepileptic events, of which 13 were psychogenic[53]

2. *What is the risk of recurrence?*

   The algorithm for decision making in an elderly patient with the first seizure is not different from younger adults.[54] Higher risk is associated with remote symptomatic etiology, interictal EEG abnormalities, focal seizures, neurological deficits, and with first seizure in sleep. Age itself is not an independent risk factor for recurrence after first seizure.[54] The proportion of provoking factors and underlying etiologies would be different. Imaging and EEG monitoring become mandatory in late onset seizures. Unless there is a clear provoking factor, the patient would be categorized as unprovoked seizure with likely remote symptomatic etiology and AED would be started.

   An example of acute symptomatic versus remote symptomatic would be an ischemic stroke. The risk of post-stroke epilepsy (remote symptomatic seizures) following an ischemic stroke is 5–9%, but the risk increases to 35% for those who had an acute symptomatic seizure at time of initial stroke.[20] A more recent multistate population-based retrospective cohort study found that about 10% of patients with stroke will develop seizures within a decade with higher risk for those with hemorrhagic stroke, nonwhite race and younger age[55]

3. *When would it be safer to withdraw the AED?*

   This is determined by similar factors as discussed under risk of recurrence. In general, unless the seizure was clearly acute symptomatic, it is safer to continue AED.

Which AED to Use?

Newer versus Older AED

The newer AEDs have some advantages over older in terms of adverse effect profile and potential for drug interactions. The major advantages of the older AEDs are efficacy and lower cost (Table 3).[56]

Each of the newer AED has some specific advantages and disadvantages that need to be considered (Table 4).[56]

A guide to selection of AED based on common comorbid conditions is presented in Table 5.

Approach to Nonconvulsive Status Epilepticus in Elderly

This requires separate mention as nonconvulsive status epilepticus (NCSE) can be a presenting event in elderly and

TABLE 3: Advantages and disadvantages of older antiepileptic drugs for elderly.

Antiepileptic drugs	Advantages	Disadvantages
Phenobarbital	Broad spectrum, once daily, cheapest	Sedation, cognitive impairment, behavioral problems, enzyme induction, bone loss
Phenytoin	Once daily, cheap	Sedation, allergic reactions, saturation kinetics, enzyme induction, bone loss
Carbamazepine	Studied in elderly, relatively cheap	Neurotoxicity, allergic reactions, enzyme inducer, hyponatremia, bone loss
Sodium valproate	Broad spectrum, a few interactions, relatively cheap	Tremor, weight gain, Parkinsonism, bone loss

TABLE 4: Advantages and disadvantages of newer antiepileptic drugs in elderly.

Antiepileptic drugs	Advantages	Disadvantages
Lamotrigine	Broad spectrum, good tolerability, a few interactions, studied in elderly	Slow titration, dose-related rash, insomnia
Gabapentin	No allergic reactions, no interactions, studied in elderly	Sedation, dizziness, weight gain
Topiramate	Broad spectrum, weight loss	Slow titration, cognitive impairment, renal stones, a few data in elderly
Oxcarbazepine	Good tolerability	Neurotoxicity, allergic rash, selective enzyme induction, hyponatremia
Tiagabine	A few allergic reactions, a few interactions	Dizziness, a few data in elderly
Levetiracetam	A few allergic reactions, no interactions	Sedation, behavioral problems
Pregabalin	No allergic reactions, no interactions	Dizziness, weight gain, a few data in elderly
Zonisamide	Broad spectrum, once daily, no interactions	Slow titration, sedation, renal stones, a few data in elderly

cannot be identified unless there is a high index of suspicion. Any elderly patient presenting with recent onset of alteration of sensorium or behavioral change should undergo EEG monitoring. NCSE should be considered in patients with

TABLE 5: Selection of antiepileptic drugs (AEDs) based on comorbid conditions—a guide.

Comorbid condition	AED to consider	AED to avoid
Obesity	Topiramate, zonisamide	Valproate (and also gabapentin, pregabalin)
Dementia, cognitive problems	–	Topiramate
Bipolar disorder	Carbamazepine, lamotrigine, valproate	–
Depression	Lamotrigine	Levetiracetam, phenobarbital
Anxiety	Gabapentin, pregabalin	Levetiracetam
Headache/migraine	Topiramate, valproate	–
Restless legs	Gabapentin	–
Osteoporosis	–	Phenobarbital, phenytoin (and carbamazepine)
Renal stones	–	Topiramate, zonisamide
Hyponatremia	–	Oxcarbazepine more than carbamazepine
Severe prior rash	–	Carbamazepine, lamotrigine, phenytoin (phenobarbital, oxcarbazepine, zonisamide)
Neutropenia, thrombocytopenia	–	Carbamazepine, phenytoin, ethosuximide, valproate
Cancer on treatment	–	Hepatic P450 enzyme inducing AED

known metabolic diseases likely to cause encephalopathy, if the degree of encephalopathy is disproportionate to the current metabolic abnormality. Finally, a patient with prolonged postictal confusion should also be screened for NCSE. A study of 236 patients with coma and no overt seizure activity found that 8% of these patients had NCSE.[57]

CONCLUSION

Both seizures and epilepsy are more common in elderly. Diagnosis can be a challenge as seizures can masquerade as dementia or behavioral change while syncope and other nonepileptic events can mimic seizures. Pharmacotherapy with AED in the elderly requires careful evaluation of quality of life, comorbidities and comedications besides chronological age. Newer AEDs provide greater options for tailoring AEDs to comorbidities but are more expensive than older AEDs.

REFERENCES

1. Ramsay RE, Rowan AJ, Pryor FM. Special considerations in treating the elderly patient with epilepsy. Neurology. 2004;62(5 Suppl 2):S24-9.
2. Sander JW, Hart YM, Johnson AL, et al. National General Practice Study of Epilepsy: newly diagnosed epileptic seizures in a general population. Lancet. 1990;336(8726):1267-71.
3. Hauser WA, Kurland LT. The epidemiology of epilepsy in Rochester, Minnesota, 1935 through 1967. Epilepsia. 1975;16(1):1-66.
4. Hauser WA. Seizure disorders: the changes with age. Epilepsia. 1992;33(Suppl 4):S6-14.
5. Hauser WA, Annegers JF, Kurland LT. Incidence of epilepsy and unprovoked seizures in Rochester, Minnesota: 1935-1984. Epilepsia. 1993;34(3):453-68.
6. Lühdorf K, Jensen LK, Plesner AM. Epilepsy in the elderly: incidence, social function, and disability. Epilepsia. 1986;27(2):135-41.
7. Tchalla AE, Marin B, Mignard C, et al. Newly diagnosed epileptic seizures: focus on an elderly population on the French island of Réunion in the Southern Indian Ocean. Epilepsia. 2011;52(12):2203-8.
8. Faught E, Richman J, Martin R, et al. Incidence and prevalence of epilepsy among older US Medicare beneficiaries. Neurology. 2012;78(7):448-53.
9. Choi H, Pack A, Elkind MSV, et al. Predictors of incident epilepsy in older adults: The Cardiovascular Health Study. Neurology. 2017;88(9):870-7.
10. Loiseau J, Loiseau P, Duché B, et al. A survey of epileptic disorders in southwest France: seizures in elderly patients. Ann Neurol. 1990;27(3):232-7.
11. Annegers JF, Hauser WA, Lee JR, et al. Incidence of acute symptomatic seizures in Rochester, Minnesota, 1935-1984. Epilepsia. 1995;36(4):327-33.
12. Stephen LJ, Brodie MJ. Epilepsy in elderly people. Lancet. 2000;355(9213):1441-6.
13. Hart YM, Sander JW, Johnson AL, et al. National General Practice Study of Epilepsy: recurrence after a first seizure. Lancet. 1990;336(8726):1271-4.
14. Roberts MA, Godfrey JW, Caird FI. Epileptic seizures in the elderly: I. Aetiology and type of seizure. Age Ageing. 1982;11(1):24-8.
15. Scarmeas N, Honig LS, Choi H, et al. Seizures in Alzheimer disease: who, when, and how common? Arch Neurol. 2009;66(8):992-7.
16. Imfeld P, Bodmer M, Schuerch M, et al. Seizures in patients with Alzheimer's disease or vascular dementia: a population-based nested case-control analysis. Epilepsia. 2013;54(4):700-7.
17. Vossel KA, Tartaglia MC, Nygaard HB, et al. Epileptic activity in Alzheimer's disease: causes and clinical relevance. Lancet Neurol. 2017;16(4):311-22.
18. Ali S, Khan MA, Khealani B. Limb-shaking Transient Ischemic Attacks: case report and review of literature. BMC Neurol. 2006;6:5.
19. Persoon S, Kappelle LJ, Klijn CJM. Limb-shaking transient ischaemic attacks in patients with internal carotid artery occlusion: a case-control study. Brain J Neurol. 2010;133(Pt 3):915-22.
20. So EL, Annegers JF, Hauser WA, et al. Population-based study of seizure disorders after cerebral infarction. Neurology. 1996;46(2):350-5.
21. Butler CR, Graham KS, Hodges JR, et al. The syndrome of transient epileptic amnesia. Ann Neurol. 2007;61(6):587-98.
22. Lee H, Yi HA, Lee SR, et al. Drop attacks in elderly patients secondary to otologic causes with Meniere's syndrome or non-Meniere peripheral vestibulopathy. J Neurol Sci. 2005;232(1–2):71-6.

23. Brantberg K, Ishiyama A, Baloh RW. Drop attacks secondary to superior canal dehiscence syndrome. Neurology. 2005;64(12):2126-8.
24. Duncan R, Oto M, Martin E, et al. Late onset psychogenic nonepileptic attacks. Neurology. 2006;66(11):1644-7.
25. Hiyoshi T, Yagi K. Epilepsy in the elderly. Epilepsia. 2000;41(Suppl 9):31-5.
26. Loiseau J, Crespel A, Picot MC, et al. Idiopathic generalized epilepsy of late onset. Seizure. 1998;7(6):485-7.
27. Rowan AJ, Ramsay RE, Collins JF, et al. New onset geriatric epilepsy: a randomized study of gabapentin, lamotrigine, and carbamazepine. Neurology. 2005;64(11):1868-73.
28. Ramsay RE, Pryor F. Epilepsy in the elderly. Neurology. 2000;55(5 Suppl 1):S9-14.
29. Theodore WH. The postictal state: effects of age and underlying brain dysfunction. Epilepsy Behav. 2010;19(2):118-20.
30. Schmucker DL. Aging and drug disposition: an update. Pharmacol Rev. 1985;37(2):133-48.
31. Lackner TE, Cloyd JC, Thomas LW, et al. Antiepileptic drug use in nursing home residents: effect of age, gender, and comedication on patterns of use. Epilepsia. 1998;39(10):1083-7.
32. Goa KL, Sorkin EM. Gabapentin: A review of its pharmacological properties and clinical potential in epilepsy. Drugs. 1993;46(3):409-27.
33. Faught E. Pharmacokinetic considerations in prescribing antiepileptic drugs. Epilepsia. 2001;42 Suppl 4:19-23.
34. Perucca E, Berlowitz D, Birnbaum A, et al. Pharmacological and clinical aspects of antiepileptic drug use in the elderly. Epilepsy Res. 2006;68 Suppl 1:S49-63.
35. Helling DK, Lemke JH, Semla TP, et al. Medication use characteristics in the elderly: the Iowa 65+ Rural Health Study. J Am Geriatr Soc. 1987;35(1):4-12.
36. Patsalos PN, Perucca E. Clinically important drug interactions in epilepsy: interactions between antiepileptic drugs and other drugs. Lancet Neurol. 2003;2(8):473-81.
37. Ensrud KE, Blackwell TL, Mangione CM, et al. Central nervous system-active medications and risk for falls in older women. J Am Geriatr Soc. 2002;50(10): 1629-37.
38. Vestergaard P, Tigaran S, Rejnmark L, et al. Fracture risk is increased in epilepsy. Acta Neurol Scand. 1999;99(5):269-75.
39. Pack AM. The Association between Antiepileptic Drugs and Bone Disease. Epilepsy Curr. 2003;3(3):91-5.
40. Sato Y, Kondo I, Ishida S, et al. Decreased bone mass and increased bone turnover with valproate therapy in adults with epilepsy. Neurology. 2001;57(3):445-9.
41. Kim SH, Lee JW, Choi KG, et al. A 6-month longitudinal study of bone mineral density with antiepileptic drug monotherapy. Epilepsy Behav. 2007;10(2):291-5.
42. Pack AM, Morrell MJ, Marcus R, et al. Bone mass and turnover in women with epilepsy on antiepileptic drug monotherapy. Ann Neurol. 2005;57(2):252-7.
43. Arora E, Singh H, Gupta YK. Impact of antiepileptic drugs on bone health: Need for monitoring, treatment, and prevention strategies. J Fam Med Prim Care. 2016;5(2):248-53.
44. Busch RM, Lineweaver TT, Naugle RI, et al. ApoE-epsilon4 is associated with reduced memory in long-standing intractable temporal lobe epilepsy. Neurology. 2007;68(6):409-14.
45. Gaitatzis A, Carroll K, Majeed A, et al. The epidemiology of the comorbidity of epilepsy in the general population. Epilepsia. 2004;45(12):1613-22.
46. Téllez-Zenteno JF, Matijevic S, Wiebe S. Somatic comorbidity of epilepsy in the general population in Canada. Epilepsia. 2005;46(12):1955-62.
47. Lühdorf K, Jensen LK, Plesner AM. Epilepsy in the elderly: prognosis. Acta Neurol Scand. 1986;74(5):409-15.
48. Brodie MJ, Overstall PW, Giorgi L. Multicentre, double-blind, randomised comparison between lamotrigine and carbamazepine in elderly patients with newly diagnosed epilepsy. The UK Lamotrigine Elderly Study Group. Epilepsy Res. 1999;37(1):81-7.

49. McIntosh S, Da Costa D, Kenny RA. Outcome of an integrated approach to the investigation of dizziness, falls and syncope in elderly patients referred to a "syncope" clinic. Age Ageing. 1993;22(1):53-8.
50. Spiegel DR, Smith J, Wade RR, et al. Transient global amnesia: current perspectives. Neuropsychiatr Dis Treat. 2017;13:2691-703.
51. Bocos-Portillo J, Escalza-Cortina I, Gómez-Beldarrain M, et al. Unilateral or bilateral punctate hippocampal hyperintensities on DW-MRI: seizures, amnesia, or both? Neurol Sci. 2018;39(9):1647-9.
52. Tatum WO, Ross J, Cole AJ. Epileptic pseudodementia. Neurology. 1998;50(5):1472-5.
53. McBride AE, Shih TT, Hirsch LJ. Video-EEG monitoring in the elderly: a review of 94 patients. Epilepsia. 2002;43(2):165-9.
54. Lawn N, Kelly A, Dunne J, et al. First seizure in the older patient: clinical features and prognosis. Epilepsy Res. 2013;107(1–2):109-14.
55. Merkler AE, Gialdini G, Lerario MP, et al. Population-based assessment of the long-term risk of seizures in survivors of stroke. Stroke. 2018;49(6):1319-24.
56. Brodie MJ, Kwan P. Epilepsy in elderly people. BMJ. 2005;331(7528):1317-22.
57. Towne AR, Waterhouse EJ, Boggs JG, et al. Prevalence of nonconvulsive status epilepticus in comatose patients. Neurology. 2000;54(2):340-5.

8

CHAPTER

Use of Antiepileptic Drugs in Pregnancy and Lactation

Ashish Bagdi

INTRODUCTION

Epilepsy affects approximately 1% of population.

Women of childbearing age constitute between 25% and 40% of all patients with epilepsy.[1,2] Approximately, 1 in 200 pregnancies is to women with epilepsy (WWE) taking antiepileptic drugs (AEDs).

Women with epilepsy have complex and multifaceted health issues.

Women with epilepsy have lower fertility rates than that of women in general population. Many AEDs interfere with efficacy of hormonal contraceptives. All major AEDs in common use have been associated with major and minor congenital malformations in developing fetus in addition they may result in intrauterine growth retardation and postnatal developmental delay.[3]

However, majority of pregnancies in WWE are uneventful.

Aim of antiepileptic therapy is to avoid convulsive seizures that are harmful for both mother and child while minimizing risks from the treatment of epilepsy.

Contraception

There is a high-unplanned pregnancy rate in WWE due to interaction between hormonal contraceptives and enzyme-inducing AEDs resulting in decreased efficacy in preventing pregnancy.

In presence of enzyme-inducing AEDs (phenytoin, phenobarbitone, carbamazepine, oxcarbazepine), it may be necessary to use oral pills with more than 50 μg of estrogen.

Planning Pregnancy in WWE

It is recommended to give folic acid in dose of 0.4 mg in all women of childbearing age because studies have found a higher mean IQ in children whose mothers receive at least 0.4 mg of folic acid periconceptionally as compared to controls.[4]

The periconceptional folate supplementation reduces the risk of neural tube defect (NTD) in children born to the women in general population.[5] In the US and Canada, folic acid fortification in cereal grains has significantly decreased the rates of NTDs.

Antiepileptic drugs alter folate metabolism and this results in congenital malformations in developing fetus.

Role of folic acid in preventing major congenital malformation (MCM) is mixed.

Hernandez et al. in a case-control study found no reduction in risk among pregnant WWE, who received folic acid supplementation.[6]

In a prospective study done in UK by Morrow, no reduction in MCM in women who take folic acid was found.[7]

Ideally, if a WWE is planning pregnancy, the neurophysician should reduce the dose of AED to the lowest effective dosage, especially in patient who is on AED with higher teratogenic risk.

If a WWE plans her pregnancy in consultation with a neurophysician then:

- Valproic acid may be avoided in the 1st trimester
- She has more chance to be on monotherapy
- She has less chances of getting seizures during pregnancy.

Adverse Effects of Seizures on Fetus and Mother and Change in Seizure Frequency during Pregnancy

Seizures during pregnancy result in adverse pregnancy outcomes.

In a study done in Taiwan by Chen et al., it was found that seizures during pregnancy increased the risk of low-birth weight infants, preterm delivery and small for gestational age births. Small for gestational age births were significantly increased in women who had seizures during pregnancy as compared to WWE who do not have seizures during pregnancy.[8]

Estrogen is proconvulsant, whereas progesterone has anticonvulsant properties.

Seizure frequency can increase or decrease during pregnancy.

In WWE who become pregnant, 17.3% experience an increase in seizure frequency and 15.9% experience a decrease in seizure frequency.[9]

The increased seizures during pregnancy have many causes like increased estrogen, increased salt and water retention, altered plasma protein binding, lack of sleep and poor compliance with the drugs.

Majority of WWE (67%) remain seizure free during pregnancy. WWE who had idiopathic generalized seizures are more likely to be seizure free than WWE who had localization-related epilepsies.[10]

About 1% of WWE may experience status epilepticus during pregnancy.

If WWE had active seizures within 1 year prior to their pregnancy, there are increased chances of intrapartum and postpartum seizures; on the contrary, if WWE are seizure free for 1 year prior to their pregnancies, there is 50–70% less risk of seizures during pregnancy.[11]

The maternal mortality rate from epilepsy is reported as 0.61 per 100,000 pregnancies.

Single most important cause of death in mothers with epilepsy is sudden unexpected death in epilepsy (SUDEP) followed by aspiration of gastric content during seizures followed by death due to drowning while taking bath.[12]

RISK OF CONGENITAL MALFORMATION WITH THE USE OF AED

The AED use during pregnancy may adversely affect the developing fetus in the following ways.

Major Congenital Malformation

These malformations result from impairment of the development of major anatomic structures and significantly affect their functioning.

These abnormalities require medical or surgical intervention or are of cosmetic importance.

Major malformations include orofacial clefts, congenital heart disease, NTD and urogenital defects (glandular hypospadias).[13]

Most common congenital malformations observed secondary to exposure to AED are cardiac malformations, hypospadias and facial clefts, respectively, which are similar to pattern of congenital malformation in general population.

Risk of congenital malformation in newborn is three times higher in WWE as compared to births given by healthy mothers (Table 1).

The risk of congenital malformations is highest with use of valproate, the risk increases with use of polytherapy (more the number of drugs used to control maternal seizures more is the risk of congenital malformations).[14]

The risk is highest in first trimester during period of organogenesis.

TABLE 1: Risk of congenital malformations associated with use of various antiepileptic drugs.

Drug	Risk of major congenital malformation	Malformations
Sodium valproate	9.3%	Neural tube defects, (spina bifida), hypospadias, cardiac defects, oral clefts
Phenobarbitone	5.5%	Cardiac defects, oral clefts, hypospadias
Topiramate	4.2%	Cleft lip, hypospadias, cardiovascular anomalies
Carbamazepine	3.0%	Neural tube defects, cardiovascular anomalies, oral clefts, hypospadias
Phenytoin	2.9%	Digital hypoplasia, cardiovascular anomalies, oral clefts
Levetiracetam	2.4%	Neural tube defects, cardiovascular anomalies
Lamotrigine	2.0%	Neural tube defects, cardiovascular anomalies

As mentioned above, use of valproate is associated with highest risk of congenital malformations in the developing fetus with 6–14% risk of malformation in born child.

With valproate, a dose response effect is demonstrated and total daily dose of 800 mg of valproate is associated with a lower risk of congenital malformation, whereas, a total dose exceeding 1,500 mg is associated with a much higher risk of malformations.[15]

To avoid fluctuations in valproate levels and to maintain a steady blood level in pregnancy, dosage of valproate may be divided into three times per day or an extended release formulation may be used.

Valproate exposure is associated with increased risk of NTDs, skeletal abnormalities (radial aplasia), urogenital defects (hypospadias), cardiovascular malformations and clefting abnormalities.[16,17]

With first trimester exposure of valproate, the risk of NTDs increases from 1 per 1,000 to 10 per 1,000 births.

Greater risk of NTDs is associated with use of valproate and carbamazepine.

Exposure to phenytoin and phenobarbitone is associated with increased risk of congenital cardiac defects and facial clefts.

Phenobarbitone use is associated with higher risk of cardiovascular malformations. A daily dose of more than 60 mg is associated with increased risk of congenital malformations. Risk of congenital malformation with use of phenobarbitone is approximately 5.5%.

The risk of oral clefts is higher with exposure to phenobarbitone, valproate and topiramate.

Exposure to topiramate is associated with higher risk of cleft palate.[18]

As per UK registry, the malformation rates with exposure to oxcarbazepine are 2.4%, with carbamazepine 2.3% and with lamotrigine 2.1%.

With lamotrigine, the risk of malformation is similar to that observed in general population.[19] Lamotrigine specifically is associated with increased risk of cleft lip and cleft palate. WWE taking less than 200 mg of lamotrigine per day have a lower risk of congenital malformation in the baby.

In general, the drugs which are associated with low frequency of seizures in WWE like valproate and phenobarbitone are associated with increased risk of congenital malformations in the fetus.[20]

On the other hand, newer antiepileptics like lamotrigine are associated with less congenital malformations but have poorer seizure control.[21]

When polytherapy is needed to control maternal seizures, it has been found that in polytherapy containing valproate, 12.5% of pregnancies were affected with a MCM, whereas only 2.7% of pregnancies were affected when polytherapy did not contain valproate.[22]

A high-quality ultrasound is recommended between 18 and 20 weeks of gestation to screen for fetal structural anomalies.

Maternal serum alpha-fetoprotein between 15 and 22 weeks of gestation combined with ultrasonography can detect up to 95% cases of fetal open NTDs.

Minor Congenital Malformations (Anomalies)

These are deviations from normal development, which do not cause a significant impairment or disability.

Examples of these anomalies are hypertelorism, acral hypoplasia of nails, etc.

Minor anomalies are two times more common in children born to WWE as compared to children born to normal mothers.

Neurodevelopmental Delay

Prenatal exposure to valproate has been associated with neurodevelopmental delay and autism.[23]

In the NEAD study, it was observed that children who have intrauterine exposure to valproate have their mean IQ 8–11 points lower at age of 6 years as compared to children who have been exposed to phenytoin, lamotrigine and carbamazepine.[24]

A lower verbal IQ is independently associated with five or more seizures in mother during pregnancy.

MECHANISMS BY WHICH AED INDUCE TERATOGENICITY

Formation of Toxic Reactive Intermediaries

Epoxide compounds formed during metabolism of AED are potentially toxic to fetal cells.

These are metabolized by enzyme epoxide hydrolase.

Phenytoin and carbamazepine give rise to epoxide metabolites.

Valproate inhibits enzyme epoxide hydrolase resulting in increased malformations in the fetus.[25]

Folate Deficiency

Folic acid is essential for DNA formation, DNA methylation and maintenance of integrity of DNA.[26]

Folate deficiency can be induced by AED administration in WWE.

Folate deficiency may induce increased plasma and tissue homocysteine levels, which may result in increased fetal malformations.[27]

Embryonic Cardiac Arrhythmias

Antiepileptic drugs such as phenytoin, phenobarbitone, carbamazepine and trimethadione may induce episodes of embryonic cardiac arrhythmias resulting in tissue hypoxia. This is followed by reoxygenation and formation of reactive oxygen species, which cause tissue damage.[28]

Induction of Apoptosis

Apoptosis or programmed cell death is induced in neurons of developing fetus by several AED like valproate, phenytoin, phenobarbitone, vigabatrin, clonazepam and diazepam.

Hence, these drugs affect fetal brain development (Table 2).

These AEDs suppress the endogenous neuroprotective systems thereby inducing apoptosis.[29]

TABLE 2: Fetal syndromes associated with antiepileptic drug.

Fetal hydantoin syndrome	Midfacial hypoplasia with a snub nose, broad nasal bridge, arched upper lip, ocular hypertelorism, hypoplasia of distal phalanges and nails
Fetal valproate syndrome	Posterior neural tube defects, upward slanting palpebral fissures, epicanthal folds, posteriorly rotated ears
Fetal phenobarbitone syndrome	Nail hypoplasia, midface hypoplasia, depressed nasal bridge, epicanthal folds, ocular hypertelorism

Genetic Susceptibility

The WWE who are homozygous for the C677T variant of the *MTHFR* gene are more likely to have fetus having fetal anticonvulsant syndromes.[30]

Genetic differences in folate metabolism may result in increased incidence of NTD in developing fetus in WWE.

Potency of antioxidant enzymes, which reduce the formation of reactive oxygen species, can be influenced by genetic differences.

BREASTFEEDING

Breastfeeding has many advantages for the newborn baby as well as the feeding mother.

For the infant, breastfeeding provides nutrition and protection against infectious diseases (by transfer of maternal antibodies), it also promotes development and psychological attachment in the infant.

Breastfeeding reduces risk of ovarian and breast cancer in the lactating mother.[31]

Most AEDs are considered safe or moderately safe during breastfeeding. However, there are certain considerations regarding AED use during lactation.

Highly protein-bound drugs like valproate, phenytoin and carbamazepine are secreted in low concentration in breast milk (clinically insignificant).

On the other hand, less protein-bound drugs such as phenobarbitone and primidone are secreted in relatively higher amounts.[32]

Please refer to Table 3 for AEDs in breast milk as a proportion of blood levels.

Infants whose mothers are on phenobarbitone or primidone may develop excessive drowsiness, poor feeding and hence

TABLE 3: Antiepileptic drugs (AEDs) in breast milk as a proportion of blood levels.

AED	Proportion appearing in breast milk
Valproic acid	<10%
Phenytoin	20%
Carbamazepine	40%
Phenobarbitone	50%
Zonisamide	41–57%
Lamotrigine	61%
Primidone	80%
Oxcarbazepine	80%
Topiramate	86%

may have poor weight gain. In such infants, serum AED level monitoring is warranted.

Following observations have been made regarding AED risk in a lactating mother:

- Use of carbamazepine, phenytoin and valproic acid is considered safe during lactation.

  Phenobarbitone and primidone can be used if combined with serum drug monitoring as and when indicated
- Gabapentin, lamotrigine, levetiracetam, oxcarbazepine, pregabalin and vigabatrin should be used in lowest possible doses.

  It is advisable to check platelet count in infants whose mother is on lamotrigine to rule out presence of thrombocytopenia[33]
- Ethosuximide is contraindicated during lactation[34]
- Zonisamide and continuous use of clonazepam and diazepam are also contraindicated during breastfeeding.

Risk of Neonatal Bleeding (Hemorrhagic Disease of the Newborn)

Neonatal bleeding has been reported in newborns of mother who have taken enzyme-inducing AEDs like phenytoin, carbamazepine and phenobarbital during pregnancy.[35]

Hence, it is advised to give mothers who are on enzyme-inducing AED 10 mg/day of oral vitamin K from 36 weeks of gestation till delivery.

Infants of such mothers are given parenteral 1 mg of vitamin K at the time of birth.[36]

AED Drug Level Monitoring

Total AED levels fall during pregnancy, but the free levels (nonprotein bound) are more or less constant.

The same dose of AED, which is used during 3rd trimester of pregnancy, needs to be continued during first 3 months postpartum.

Lamotrigine levels can fall precipitously during 3rd trimester of pregnancy due to enzyme induction.[37] Hence, its dose may have to be increased during the 3rd trimester.

Metabolism rate of levetiracetam increases during pregnancy.[37]

A baseline preconceptional free AED level repeated during beginning of each trimester and last 4 weeks of pregnancy is sufficient in a woman whose seizures are fairly well controlled.

Additional AED levels may be done when seizures are poorly controlled or when there is concern about the noncompliance.

CONCLUSION

- Prenatal counseling is advised to all WWE.
- They must be informed that majority of pregnancies in WWE are uneventful.
- They must be informed about the risk of teratogenicity with the use of AED.
- If patient come well in advance before pregnancy, the use of valproate should be avoided in view of high teratogenicity and risk of neurodevelopmental delay in children who were exposed to valproate in utero. Lamotrigine is a good alternative to valproate.
- Women with localization-related epilepsy should be treated with carbamazepine.
- Five milligram of folate per day is recommended to prevent NTDs.
- Prenatal ultrasonography and serum alpha-fetoprotein levels must be done as recommended to screen for congenital malformations and NTDs, respectively.
- Free AED drug levels should be done as recommended and to check for compliance.
- Pregnant women who are on enzyme-inducing AED should be given vitamin K in recommended doses to prevent hemorrhagic disease of the newborn.
- Breastfeeding is considered safe in WWE who are on AED.
- Lastly, in WWE, those who have uncontrolled seizures, higher potency AEDs use is warranted, but these drugs have higher risk of inducing congenital malformations in the developing fetus.
- On the other hand, if seizures are well under control then these WWE can be managed with the lowest possible dose of AED.
- As far as possible, polytherapy should be avoided.
- Hence, a balance should be maintained between seizure control and risk of congenital malformations, while using AED.

REFERENCES

1. Kinney MO, Craig JJ. Pregnancy and epilepsy: meeting the challenges over the last 25 years: the rise of the pregnancy registries. Seizure. 2017;44:162-8.
2. Chen YH, Chiou HY, Lin HC, et al. Effect of seizures during gestation on pregnancy outcomes in women with epilepsy. Arch Neurol. 2009;66:979-84.
3. Tomson T, Perucca E, Battino D. Navigating toward fetal and maternal health: the challenge of treating epilepsy in pregnancy. Epilepsia. 2004;45:1171-5.
4. Meador KJ, Baker GA, Browning N, et al. Fetal antiepileptic drug exposure and cognitive outcomes at age 6 years (NEAD study): a prospective observational study. Lancet Neurol. 2013;12:244-52.
5. Morrow JI, Craig JJ. Anti-epileptic drugs in pregnancy: current safety and other issues. Expert Opin Pharmacother. 2003;4:445-56.

6. Hernandez-Diaz S, Werler MM, Walker AM, et al. Folic acid antagonists during pregnancy and the risk of birth defects. N Engl J Med. 2000;343:1608-14.
7. Morrow JI, Hunt SJ, Russell AJ, et al. Folic acid use and major congenital malformations in offspring of women with epilepsy: a prospective study from the UK Epilepsy and Pregnancy Register. J Neurol Neurosurg Psychiatr. 2009;80: 506-11.
8. Chen YH, Chiou HY, Lin HC, et al. Effect of seizures during gestation on pregnancy outcomes in women with epilepsy. Arch Neurol. 2009;66:979-84.
9. EURAP Study Group. Seizure control and treatment in pregnancy: observations from the EURAP epilepsy pregnancy registry. Neurology. 2006;66:354-60.
10. Battino D, Tomson T, Bonizzoni E, et al. Seizure control and treatment changes in pregnancy: observations from the EURAP epilepsy pregnancy registry. Epilepsia. 2013;54:1621-7.
11. Vajda FJ, Hitchcock A, Graham J, et al. Seizure control in antiepileptic drug-treated pregnancy. Epilepsia. 2008;49:172-6.
12. Kapoor D, Wallace S. Trends in maternal deaths from epilepsy in the United Kingdom: a 30-year retrospective review. Obstet Med. 2014;7:160-4.
13. Holmes LB. Need for inclusion and exclusion criteria for the structural abnormalities recorded in children born from exposed pregnancies. Teratology. 1999;59:1-2.
14. Meador K, Reynolds MW, Crean S, et al. Pregnancy outcomes in women with epilepsy: A systematic review and meta-analysis of published pregnancy registries and cohorts. Epilepsy Res. 2008;81:1-13.
15. Tomson T, Battino D, Bonizzoni E, et al. Dose-dependent risk of malformations with antiepileptic drugs: an analysis of data from the EURAP epilepsy and pregnancy registry. Lancet Neurol. 2011;10:609-17.
16. Campbell E, Kennedy F, Russell A, et al. Malformation risks of antiepileptic drug monotherapies in pregnancy: updated results from the UK and Ireland Epilepsy and Pregnancy Registers. J Neurol Neurosurg Psychiatry. 2014;85:1029-34.
17. Jentink J, Loane MA, Dolk H, et al. Valproic acid monotherapy in pregnancy and major congenital malformations. N Engl J Med. 2010;362:2185-93.
18. Peller A, Westgate MN, Holmes L. Trends in congenital malformations, 1974–1999: effect of prenatal diagnosis and elective termination. Obstet Gynecol. 2004;104:957-64.
19. Cunnington M, Tennis P; International Lamotrigine Pregnancy registry Scientific Advisory Committee. Lamotrigine and the risk of malformations in pregnancy. Neurology. 2005;64:955-60.
20. Hernandez-Diaz S, Smith CR, Shen A, et al. Comparative safety of antiepileptic drugs during pregnancy. Neurology. 2012;78:1692-9.
21. Vajda F, Lander C, O'Brien T, et al. Australian Pregnancy Registry of Women Taking Antiepileptic Drugs. Epilepsia. 2004;45:1466.
22. Cunnington M, Tennis P. Lamotrigine and the risk of malformations in pregnancy. Neurology. 2005;64:955-60.
23. Dean J, Hailey H, Moore S, et al. Long term health and neurodevelopment in children exposed to antiepileptic drugs before birth. J Med Genetics. 2002;39:251-9.
24. Meador KJ, Baker GA, Browning N, et al. Fetal antiepileptic drug exposure and cognitive outcomes at age 6 years (NEAD study): a prospective observational study. Lancet Neurol. 2013;12:244-52.
25. Lindhout D, Hoppener RJ, Meinardi H. Teratogenicity of antiepileptic drug combinations with special emphasis on epoxidation (of carbamazepine). Epilepsia. 1984;25:77-83.
26. Lavoie A, Tripp E, Parsa K, et al. Polyglutamate forms of folate in resting and proliferating mammalian tissues. Clin Sci Mol Med. 1975;48:67-73.
27. Gos MJ, Szpecht-Potocka A. Genetic basis of neural tube defects. II. Genes correlated with folate and methionine metabolism. J Appl Genet. 2002;43:511-24.
28. Azarbayjani F, Danielsson BR. Embryonic arrhythmia by inhibition of HERG channels: A common hypoxia-related teratogenic mechanism for antiepileptic drugs? Epilepsia. 2002;43:457-68.

29. Bittigau P, Sifringer M, Genz K, et al. Antiepileptic drugs and apoptotic neurodegeneration in the developing brain. Proc Natl Acad Sci U S A. 2002;99:15089-94.
30. Dean JC, Moore SJ, Osborne A, et al. Fetal anticonvulsant syndrome and mutation in the maternal MTHFR gene. Clin Genet. 1999;56:216-20.
31. Ip S, Chung M, Raman G, et al. A summary of the Agency for Healthcare Research and Quality's evidence report on breastfeeding in developed countries. Breastfeed Med. 2009;4(suppl 1):S17-30.
32. Pennell PB. Antiepileptic drug pharmacokinetics during pregnancy and lactation. Neurology. 2003;61(6 Suppl 2):35-42.
33. Newport DJ, Pennell PB, Calamaras MR, et al. Lamotrigine in breast milk and nursing infants: determination of exposure. Pediatrics. 2008;122:e223-31.
34. Hale TW. Medications and Mother's milk 2012: A Manual of Lactational Pharmacology, 15th edition. 1712 N Forest Amarillo, TX: Hale Publishing; 2012. pp. 79106-7017; 184-6; 264-5; 325-6; 426-7; 495-6; 651-3; 664-5; 870-1; 905-6; 910-11; 938-9; 940-1; 1077; 1091-2; 1126-7; 1136-7; 1161-2.
35. Morrow JI, Craig JJ. Anti-epileptic drugs in pregnancy: current safety and other issues. Expert Opin Pharmacother. 2003;4:445-56.
36. National Institute for Clinical Excellence. The Epilepsies. The Diagnosis and Management of the Epilepsies in Adults and Children in Primary and Secondary Care. Clinical Guideline 20. London: NICE; 2012.
37. Weston J, Bromley R, Jackson CF, et al. Monotherapy treatment of epilepsy in pregnancy: congenital malformation outcomes in the child. Cochrane Database Syst Rev. 2016;11:CD010224.

9

CHAPTER

Use of Antiepileptic Drug in Systemic Disorders

Bindu Menon

USE OF ANTIEPILEPTIC DRUG IN SYSTEMIC DISORDERS

Epilepsy is a common neurological disorder affecting 1% of population. Seizures can be a part of the systemic illness, and the choice of antiepileptic drugs (AEDs) during the management in such situations can be very challenging. A major proportion of patients with epilepsy have comorbid illness. The comorbid illness influences the treatment of epilepsy. This includes decision during acute seizure management and for chronic therapy as well. The goal of epilepsy treatment is obviously complete seizure freedom improving the overall quality of life. The underlying primary organ disease, which can be cardiac, hepatic, renal, or endocrine disorders, has significant effects on metabolism, absorption, protein binding, and clearance of AEDs. The older AEDs have a high plasma protein-binding capacity. Majority of the drugs are metabolized by cytochrome P450 enzyme system in the liver and have a renal excretion.

The therapeutic drug level evaluation is necessary in cases of AED toxicity due to active secondary metabolites, which are more so common with older AEDs. The improved pharmacokinetic profile of newer AEDs gives a better treatment safety profile.

In critically ill patients, the free drug concentration tends to rise due to altered serum proteins as a result of elevated acute phase reactions and low-serum albumin (A).[1]

This chapter gives an overview of which antiepileptic to choose and the safety profile in each systemic condition.

CARDIOVASCULAR DISEASE

Several AEDs have known cardiovascular side effects and need to be used with caution. Phenytoin (PHT), a commonly used intravenous AED in the setting of acute seizure or status epilepticus, can cause hypotension and cardiac arrhythmias. This is more common, if the patient has an underlying cardiac problem or the rate of infusion is very rapid.

Phenytoin and fosphenytoin use is contraindicated in patients with severe cardiac disease and heart blocks. The intravenous infusion of phenytoin should be 10 mg/min or less with electrocardiographic and blood pressure monitoring.[2] Hence, phenytoin or fosphenytoin are not the drug of first choice in cardiac patients with epilepsy. Carbamazepine (CBZ) is known to have negative chronotropic and dromotropic effects on the conducting system.[3] Underlying cardiac diseases like cardiac conduction defects are particular risk factors.[4,5] A doubtful association between CBZ and sudden unexpected death in epilepsy (SUDEP)[6] has been suggested though it is not consistent.[7]

Valproate (VPA), a broad-spectrum AED, has 1–5% chances of inducing hypertension, tachycardia and palpitation.[8] However, VPA is relatively safe preferably with BP monitoring in acute intravenous use. The newer AED, lacosamide (LCM), has been better tolerated with minimal cardiac side effects except increased heart rate particularly with rapid high dosing.[9] Lacosamide should be used with caution in patients with cardiac conduction abnormalities or drugs which prolong the PR interval.

Levetiracetam (LEV) rarely has any cardiac side effects and is suitable in emergency as well as maintenance therapy. Lamotrigine (LTG) is a safer option because of lack of enzyme-inducing properties. Table 1 shows the drugs to be used with caution in cardiac patients.

The safer AEDs in cardiac patients are LEV, LCM, topiramate (TPM), LTG, VPA and zonisamide (ZNS).

LIVER DISEASE

Metabolism of majority of AEDs occurs predominantly in the liver. In mild hepatic dysfunction, there is generally no need for AED adjustment. The hepatic metabolism and hypoalbuminemia alter the AED pharmacokinetics. Dose adjustments are generally not required in acute viral hepatitis.[10,11] Cirrhosis of liver alters the protein-binding metabolism and elimination and hence requires dose adjustment.

Antiepileptic drugs predominantly metabolized in liver are PHT, VPA, CBZ, phenobarbital (PB), benzodiazepines (BDZ), oxcarbazepine (OXC) and LTG. LEV, TPM and ZNS are partially metabolized in the liver. Gabapentin and vigabatrin are not metabolized in liver. VPA and felbamate (FBM) are to be avoided in patients with hepatic impairment. Phenytoin-free levels are increased due to hypoalbuminemia and high protein binding

TABLE 1: Drugs to be used with caution in cardiac patients.

AED	Cardiac drug	Interaction/effect
Phenytoin	Ticlopidine	Increases PHT level
	Antiarrhythmic	Increases metabolism of antiarrhythmic drugs
	Amiodarone	Increases PHT levels
	Beta-blockers	Increases β-blocker metabolism
	Dihydropyridine	Increases dihydropyridine metabolism
	Losartan	PHT reduces active metabolite by 63%
	Oral anticoagulants (OAC)	Reduces effects of OAC OAC increases PHT levels
	Diuretics	PHT reduces the diuretic response
	Digoxin	PHT reduces digoxin levels
	Statins	PHT stimulates statins metabolism
CB2	Ticlopidine	Increases the level of CB2
	Antiarrhythmic	Increases antiarrhythmic metabolism of diltiazem/verapamil increase CB2 levels
	Antihypertensive	Increases metabolism of β-blockers
	OAC	Reduces the effect of OAC
	Diuretics	Use with caution to avoid hypernatremia
	Statins	Stimulates the metabolism of statins
VPA	Salicylates	Increases the free fraction of VPA
	Antihypertensive	Increases level of nimodipine by 50%

(PHT: phenytoin; VPA: valproate)

and hence can lead to toxicity. LEV is the best alternative in acute treatment of seizures in patients with liver disease. Long-term AED treatment must be given due consideration. Most AEDs are low-extraction drugs, i.e. the extraction rate is less than 30% during first passage through liver. Hence, treatment can be initiated at regular dose with low-maintenance dose.[12]

Antiepileptic drugs with low protein binding and less hepatic metabolism like LEV, OXC and TPM are more suitable. However, in severe hepatic impairment, the doses of these safe AEDs will also need to be reduced, as there is often concomitant renal impairment. Plasma AED concentration may be done to monitor for toxicity.

Generalized or nonconvulsive status is known to occur in stage III to IV hepatic failure. Seizures could be due to increased ammonia levels or increased excitatory neurotransmitters. Initial treatment is targeted at reducing ammonia and cerebral edema. However, if these fail, AED needs to be supplemented. However, PHT and BDZ are ineffective, and BDZ produces sedation and is to be avoided. LVT is a safe alternative.[13]

RENAL DISEASE

The half-life of AEDs eliminated by kidney increases and leads to drug accumulation. The choice of AED depends on the type of seizure; however, the plasma kinetics of AED needs to be kept in mind.

Albuminuria, plasma protein binding changes, reduced glomerular filtration and tubular secretion, metabolic acidosis, and gastroparesis are some of the factors that lead to change in AED levels; drug elimination is decreased due to reduced glomerular filtration and tubular secretion. Decreased serum albumin levels due to proteinuria and metabolic acidosis also lead to decreased binding capacity leading to increased free drug levels. Toxins in uremic encephalopathy may bind to plasma proteins and hence reduced protein binding, leading to increased free AED levels in plasma.[14,15] Loading dose of AEDs may be the same as in healthy subjects; however, the maintenance doses are to be adjusted according to the creatinine clearance, and adjustments are done either by reducing the dose or increasing the interval between the doses.[16]

The AEDs eliminated by kidney like LEV, LTG, OXC, TPM and ZNS may need dose adjustment, however, are not contraindicated. TPM and ZNS should be avoided in patients with nephrolithiasis. BDZ, CBZ, ethosuximide, PHT, VPA and tiagabine (TGB) are the most recommended AEDs, which are predominantly eliminated by liver. Hydrosoluble AEDs with minimal protein binding and low-distribution volume require dose adjustment.[17] Supplementary AED doses may be required after dialysis. Fifty percent of AED loss occurs during hemodialysis with LVT, TPM and ZNS. Hence, supplementary doses are required after hemodialysis. LTG, OXC, TGB and gabapentin do not require adjustment as these drugs do not have dialysis-associated loss.

PSYCHIATRIC DISORDERS

The risk for developing seizures is more in patients with depression, and depression is also twice as common in patients with epilepsy. The coexistence of psychiatric symptoms has an impact on the treatment of epilepsy. Psychiatric comorbidity and suicidal behavior tendencies are markedly increased in patients with epilepsy. Due to the diverse mechanisms of action, AEDs broadly fall under two categories—sedating and activating group. Sedative group comprises of GABA-inhibiting drugs such as barbiturates, BDZ, valproate, gabapentin, TGB and vigabatrin. Second group is the glutamate excitatory group such as felbamate and LTG. TPM has both properties and has mixed profiles.[18] The sedative drugs, though promote sleep and have anxiolytic properties, may impair attention and induce lethargy and low mood. On the contrary, the excitatory group can induce insomnia anxiety, and agitation. LTG has positive effects on mood and antidepressant effect.[17] LEV has been associated with aggressive behavior.[19] Phenytoin and valproate are known to be associated with less irritability.[20] Antidepressants have been known to have proconvulsant effects. However, most reported seizures are noted with high doses of antidepressants.[21] A pivotal study reviewing data from the food and drug administration phases II and III found a higher incidence of seizures than the placebo included clomipramine and bupropion.[22]

The other antidepressants found to have increased incidence of seizures in a dose-dependent manner are amoxapine and maprotiline.[23] Most other antidepressants were found to be safe at therapeutic doses.

One needs to look at the synergistic side effects of AEDs and antipsychotics while treating patients with epilepsy. Weight gain needs to be considered with VPA and CBZ. Fluoxetine is usually a preferred drug with relatively less weight gain with added advantage of alerting effect. However, it increases the plasma concentrations of CBZ and PHT; hence, serum levels need to be monitored. Hyponatremia needs to be considered when serotonin and norepinephrine reuptake inhibitors (SNRIs) are used with CBZ, OXC and eslicarbazepine acetate. AEDs with negative psychotropic effects like BDZ, barbiturates, TPM, LEV and ZNS should be used with caution while LTG, LCM, pregabalin, and gabapentin have beneficial effects. Paroxetine and citalopram do not show such interaction.

Enzyme induction also plays a pivotal role while deciding the AED. First-line AEDs like CBZ, PHT and PB are potent cytochrome P450 (CYP) enzymes inducers at regular doses, while OXC and TPM induce at higher doses. This enzyme induction can reduce the serum concentration of the drugs, which have same enzyme substrates like tricyclic antidepressants (TCAs) and all selective serotonin reuptake inhibitors (SSRIs) and SNRIs. Hence, the doses of amitriptyline, nortriptyline, doxepin, clomipramine, mianserin, nomifensine, bupropion and, to a lesser extent, citalopram and paroxetine need to be increased. VPA inhibits TCA metabolism and, therefore, may increase

TABLE 2: Psychiatric medications and their level of seizure risk.

Level of risk	High risk	Medium risk	Low risk
Psychiatric medications	• Bupropion • Clomipramine, chlorpromazine, clozapine	Tricyclic antidepressants, venlafaxine, thioridazine, olanzapine, quetiapine	• Fluoxetine • Sertraline • Paroxetine • Trazodone • Haloperidol • Risperidone

TCA serum levels. The newer AEDs (LTG, TGB, LEV and ZNS) are devoid of this effect. Paroxetine and sertraline affect plasma concentrations of CBZ and PHT. VPA and LTG toxicity has been seen with sertraline doses between 25 and 100 mg. Fluoxetine increases phenytoin concentration, probably due to CYP 2C9 inhibition. Psychiatric drugs and their effect on seizures are listed in Table 2.[24]

Persons with epilepsy may be at increased risk for suicide. In 2008, the link between suicide and AEDs was highlighted with the Food and Drug Administration (FDA) issuing a warning against almost all AEDs depending on the meta-analysis of 11 AEDs from a multicenter randomized controlled study.[25] Now, even though there have been 80 publications over the last 10 years of the first FDA warning, there is lack of evidence for any particular AED.

PORPHYRIA

Porphyria is a group of diseases in which skin and nervous system are affected by abnormal accumulation of porphyrins. It is a reverse disorder of heme metabolism generalized and partial seizures are seen in 5–15% of patients.[26] Epileptic seizures are induced by most AEDs and cannot be used in chronic therapy. Acute attacks can be treated with BDZ. Gabapentin does not induce hepatic metabolism and is safe. Bromides were used in the past, however, not used now. Clonazepam has been found to be useful in a few cases. Intravenous magnesium has been used to treat status epilepticus[27] while gabapentin and LEV are used as maintenance therapy. Propofol has also been used safely in status epilepticus.[28]

EPILEPSY AND THYROID DISEASE

Antiepileptic drugs have shown to have a negative impact on the endocrine system in children and adults.[29] First-line AEDs (PHT, PB, CBZ, and VPA) and OXC are known to affect thyroid function.[30-33] A study had found that CBZ was most commonly associated with a low-thyroid hormone level, females being more affected.[34] The thyroid valves are seen to normalize after AED withdrawal.[35] Hence in patients with thyroid diseases, use of EIAED (enzyme-inducing antiepileptic drug) may be avoided. Several mechanisms have been postulated for the AED-induced thyroid changes. Enzyme induction accelerates the clearance of thyroid hormone. AED also interferes with hypothalamic–pituitary axis.[36] A study investigating the effect of CBZ, PB, OXC, LEV and VPA on thyroid function in children concluded that all AEDs except LEV, had varying degrees of deleterious effects on thyroid function.[37]

REFERENCES

1. Knake S, Hamer HM, Rosenow F. Status epilepticus: a critical review. Epilepsy Behav. 2009;15:10-14.
2. Adams BD, Buckley NH, Kim JY, et al. Fosphenytoin may cause hemodynamically unstable bradydysrhythmias. J Emerg Med. 2006;30:75-9.
3. Ide A, Kamijo Y. Intermittent complete atrioventricular block after long term low-dose carbamazepine therapy with a serum concentration less than the therapeutic level. Intern Med. 2007;46:627-9.
4. Knilans TK. Carbamazepine-induced atrioventricular block in a child with tuberous sclerosis and cardiac rhabdomyoma. Ann Neurol. 1994;36:804-5.
5. Kumada T, Hattori H, Doi H, et al. Postoperative complete atrioventricular block induced by carbamazepine in a patient with congenital heart disease. No To Hattatsu. 2005;37:257-61.
6. Timmings PL. Sudden unexpected death in epilepsy: is carbamazepine implicated? Seizure. 1998:7:289-91.
7. Hitiris N, Suratman S, Kelly K, et al. Sudden unexpected death in epilepsy: a search for risk factors. Epilepsy Behav. 2007;10:138-41.
8. Lexicomp Online. Valproic Acid and Derivatives (Pediatric & Neonatal Lexi-Drugs). Hudson, Ohio, USA: Lexi-Comp; 2015.
9. Luk ME, Tatum WO, Patel AV, et al. The Safety of lacosamide for treatment of seizures and seizure prophylaxis in adult hospitalized patients. Neurohospitalist. 2012:2:77-81.
10. Alvin J, McHorse T, Hoyumpa A, et al. The effect of liver disease in man on the disposition of phenobarbital. J Pharmacol Exp Ther. 1975;192:224-35.
11. Kraus JW, Desmond PV, Marshall JP, et al. Effects of aging and liver disease on disposition of lorazepam. Clin Pharmacol Ther. 1978;24:411-9.
12. Delco F, Tchambaz L, Schlienger R, et al. Dose adjustment in patients with liver disease. Drug Saf. 2005;28:529-45.
13. Chabolla DR, Harnois DM, Meschia JF. Levetiracetam mono-therapy for liver transplant patients with seizures. Transplant Proc. 2003;35:1480-1.
14. Gabardi S, Abramson S. Drug dosing in chronic kidney disease. Med Clin North Am. 2005;89:649-87.
15. Lacerda G, Krummel T, Sabourdy C, et al. Optimizing therapy of seizures in patients with renal or hepatic dysfunction. Neurology. 2006;67(Suppl 4):S28-S33.
16. Patsalos PN, Berry DJ, Bourgeois BF, et al. Antiepileptic drugs—best practice guidelines for therapeutic drug monitoring: a position paper by the subcommission on therapeutic drug monitoring, ILAE Commission on Therapeutic Strategies. Epilepsia. 2008;49(7):1239-76.
17. Israni RK, Kasbekar N, Haynes K, et al. Use of antiepileptic drugs in patients with kidney disease. Sem Dialysis. 2006;19:408-16.
18. Fakhoury TA, Miller JM, Hammer AE, et al. Effects of lamotrigine on mood in older adults with epilepsy and comorbid depressive symptoms: an open-label, multicentre, prospective study. Drugs Aging. 2008;25:955-62.
19. Mula M, Trimble MR, Yuen A, et al. Psychiatric adverse events during levetiracetam therapy. Neurology. 2003;61:704-6.
20. Berg I, Butler A, Ellis M, et al. Psychiatric aspects of epilepsy in childhood treated with carbamazepine, phenytoin or sodium valproate: a random trial. Dev Med Child Neurol. 1993;35:149-57.
21. Rosenstein D, Nelson J, Jacobs S. Seizures associated with antidepressants: a review. J Clin Psychiatry. 1993;54:289-99.
22. Alper K, Schwartz KA, Kolts RL, et al. Seizure incidence in psychopharmacological clinical trials: an analysis of Food and Drug Administration (FDA) summary basis of approval reports. Biol Psychiatry. 2007;62:345-54.
23. Jobe PC, Dailey JW, Wernicke JF. A noradrenergic and serotonergic hypothesis of the linkage between epilepsy and affective disorders. Crit Rev Neurobiol. 1999;13:317-56.

24. Pérez EB. Epilepsy and related psychiatric conditions. Section I: Psychiatry and Pediatrics. In: Editor Rey JM (Ed). IACAPAP Textbook of Child and Adolescent Mental Health; 2015 Edition. IACAPAP; 2015.
25. US Food and Drug Administration. (2008). Antiepileptic drugs and suicidality. [online] Available from http://www.fda.gov/ohrms/dockets/ac/08/briefing/2008-4372b1-01-FDA.pdf [Last accessed February, 2019].
26. Bylesio I, Forsgren L, Lithner F, et al. Epidemiology and clinical characteristics of seizures in patients with acute intermittent porphyria. Epilepsia. 1996;37:230-5.
27. Taylor RL. Magnesium sulfate for AIP seizures. Neurology. 1981;31:1371-2.
28. Weir PM, Hodkinson BP. Is propofol a safe agent in porphyria? Anaesthesia. 1988;43:1022-3.
29. Svalheim S, Sveberg L, Mochol M, et al. Interactions between antiepileptic drugs and hormones. Seizure. 2015;28:12-7.
30. Franklyn JA, Sheppard MC, Ramsden DB. Measurement of free thyroid hormones in patients on long-term phenytoin therapy. Eur J Clin Pharmacol. 1984;26:633-4.
31. Zhang YX, Shen CH, Lai QL, et al. Effects of antiepileptic drug on thyroid hormones in patients with epilepsy: a meta-analysis. Seizure. 2016;35:72-9.
32. Isojarvi JI, Airaksinen KE, Mustonen JN, et al. Thyroid and myocardial function after replacement of carbamazepine by oxcarbazepine. Epilepsia. 1995;36:810-6.
33. Vainionpaa LK, Mikkonen K, Rattya J, et al. Thyroid function in girls with epilepsy with carbamazepine, oxcarbazepine, or valproate monotherapy and after withdrawal of medication. Epilepsia. 2004;45:197-203.
34. Shih FY, Chuang YC, Chuang MJ, et al. Effects of antiepileptic drugs on thyroid hormone function in epilepsy patients. Seizure. 2017;48:7-10.
35. Lossius MI, Taubøll E, Mowinckel P, et al. Reversible effects of antiepileptic drugs on thyroid hormones in men and women with epilepsy: a prospective randomized double-blind withdrawal study. Epilepsy Behav. 2009;16:64-8.
36. Verrotti A, Scardapane A, Manco R, et al. Antiepileptic drugs and thyroid function. J Pediatr Endocrinol Metab. 2008;21:401-8.
37. Zhang YX, Shen CH, Lai QL, et al. Effects of antiepileptic drug on thyroid hormones in patients with epilepsy: A meta-analysis. Seizure. 2016;35:72-9.

10
CHAPTER

Drug of Choice in Various Epilepsies

Dinesh Nayak

INTRODUCTION

Epilepsy is one of the most common neurological disorders, which not only produces seizures as the main manifestation, but also has a profound impact on the psychosocial, educational and occupational domains. The treatment of epilepsy, therefore, has to take into account not just antiepileptic medication, but also ensure that the psychosocial aspects are managed, in order to obtain the best outcomes.

The cornerstone of treatment remains antiepileptic drugs (AEDs). From 1857, when bromides were introduced, until 1975, there were only six AEDs to choose from—(1) phenobarbitone (PB), (2) phenytoin (PHT), (3) primidone (PRM), (4) carbamazepine (CBZ), (5) sodium valproate (VPA) and (6) clonazepam (CLZ). These are termed "older AEDs" or the "first-generation AEDs". The last 25 years have seen an explosion of "newer AEDs", the so-called "second- and third-generation AEDs". With such a bewildering array of AEDs in the therapeutic armamentarium, it is imperative for the modern day physician to have a good understanding of the mechanism of action, pharmacokinetic and pharmacodynamic interactions, and adverse effect profile of these agents. Moreover, all the newer AEDs are two to three times more expensive than the first-generation AEDs, therefore, making them unaffordable for a significant proportion of patients.

This chapter will outline the principles of AED choice for different seizure types and epilepsy syndromes, as well as their use in special situations such as in women with epilepsy, in the elderly, and in patients with organ dysfunction. The chapter will also guide the reader on the advantages and disadvantages of the older and the newer AEDs, so as to enable them to use these drugs judiciously.

The management of epilepsy is best done in an orderly stepwise manner.

STEP 1: ACCURATE DIAGNOSIS

The diagnosis of an epileptic seizure and epilepsy is clinical, while the electroencephalography (EEG) is used mainly to support the clinical diagnosis of epilepsy, and not to exclude it. Similarly, neuroimaging cannot rule in or rule out epilepsy. Therefore, it is important for the clinician to obtain a detailed description of the evolution of symptoms and the circumstances in which they occur from the patient and the eyewitness in order to make a correct diagnosis of an epileptic seizure. A good history will help rule out many of the paroxysmal, physiological and psychological conditions that mimic epileptic seizures. The EEG is then employed to help establish an electroclinical syndromic diagnosis.

STEP 2: EPILEPSY EDUCATION

The next step is to counsel the patient and the family about the condition. It is important for the physician to make the correct diagnosis and arrive at the syndromic diagnosis. If the diagnosis is benign rolandic epilepsy, the parents can be counseled that the condition spontaneously remits by adolescence, and that AEDs may not be required for many of the patients. However, if the diagnosis is of a symptomatic generalized syndrome such as Lennox–Gastaut syndrome, the prognosis is poor and AED therapy may be have to be administered indefinitely. Educating the patient and the family members about the condition as well as the first aid during a seizure and acute care is important.

STEP 3: CHOOSING THE APPROPRIATE ANTIEPILEPTIC DRUG

Since the treatment of epilepsy is mainly based on AED therapy, which requires to be administered for several years, it is of paramount importance for the physician to choose the medication with utmost care. Choosing the right AED, be it old or new, depends on several factors, such as seizure type, epilepsy syndrome, efficacy, gender, cost, pharmacokinetic profile, adverse effects and patient comorbidities.

The first-generation (older) AEDs remain the mainstay in the treatment for majority of the population in our country. The advantages of using older AEDs are that they are effective in controlling most types of seizures, are inexpensive, and have been in use for decades, with most physicians being familiar with their use. They are also familiar with the adverse effects. They are effective in the treatment of a variety of seizures and epilepsies. The main disadvantage of the older AEDs is that they have pharmacodynamic and pharmacokinetic interactions with other medication, due to enzyme induction through their effect on the hepatic cytochrome P450 (CYP) enzyme superfamily. While most AEDs are safe during pregnancy, VPA should be avoided during pregnancy in view of high incidence of neural tube defects in the fetus.

The main advantages of the newer AEDs are that they are as efficacious as the older AEDs, are better tolerated with fewer adverse effects, and lesser enzyme induction than the older AEDs. Therefore, they have fewer pharmacodynamic and pharmacokinetic interactions with other concomitantly administered drugs. They are fairly safe during pregnancy, although data on the use of some of the newest AEDs during pregnancy is lacking. One of the biggest disadvantages of the newer AEDs is that they are at least twice as expensive as the older AEDs. This is important in our country, where patients have to spend on treatment from their pockets, and they require to be taken for several years.

Choosing the right AED, be it old or new, depends on several factors, such as seizure type, epilepsy syndrome, efficacy, gender, cost, pharmacokinetic profile, adverse effects and patient comorbid conditions.[1]

In 2008, the Indian Epilepsy Society constituted the Guidelines for Management of Epilepsy in India (GEMIND)[2] to help physicians choose the right AED for the treatment of epilepsies (Table 1). The AED choice for different seizure types is as follows:

Focal seizures: The first-generation drugs like CBZ, PHT, PB and VPA are excellent choices. Among the newer AEDs, oxcarbazepine (OXC), levetiracetam (LEV), lamotrigine (LTG), topiramate (TPM) and lacosamide (LCM) are effective.

Generalized absence seizures: Ethosuximide (ESM) and VPA among the older AEDs and LTG, TPM and CLB among the newer AEDs.

TABLE 1: Antiepileptic drugs (AEDs) choice for different seizure types.

Seizure type	First-line AEDs	Second-line AEDs
Focal seizures	CBZ, PHT, PB, VPA, CLZ	OXC, LEV, LTG, LCM, TPM, ZNS, CLB, PER
Myoclonic seizures	VPA, CLZ	LEV, TPM, ZNS, CLZ
Generalized absence seizures	ESM, VPA	LTG, TPM, CLB
Primarily generalized tonic-clonic	VPA	LEV, LTG, TPM, ZNS
Generalized after a focal onset	CBZ, PHT, PB	OXC, LEV, LTG, LCM, TPM, ZNS, CLB, PER
Atypical absence	VPA	LTG, TPM, ZNS, CLB
Drop attacks	VPA	CLB, LTG, TPM, ZNS

(CBZ: carbamazepine; PHT: phenytoin; PB: phenobarbitone; VPA: sodium valproate; ESM: ethosuximide; OXC: oxcarbazepine; LEV: levetiracetam; LTG: lamotrigine; TPM: topiramate; CLB: clobazam; ZNS: zonisamide; CLZ: clonazepam; LCM: lacosamide; PER: perampanel)

Myoclonic seizures: Sodium valproate (VPA) and CLZ among older AEDs and LEV, ZNS, TPM among the newer AEDs.

Primary generalized tonic-clonic seizures: The drug of choice is VPA. Among the newer AEDs, LEV, TPM, ZNS and LTG are good.

Generalized seizures after a focal onset: Phenytoin (PHT), PB, CBZ and valproate among the older AEDs and LEV, OXC, LTG, TPM, ZNS, LCM, CLB and perampanel (PER) among the newer AEDs.

Atypical absence: Sodium valproate (VPA) among the older AEDs, and LEV, LTG, TPM and ZNS among the newer AEDs.

Drop attacks: Sodium valproate (VPA) among the older AEDs and CLB, TPM, ZNS and LTG among the newer AEDs.

West syndrome, infantile spasms: Although adrenocorticotropic hormone (ACTH) has been the mainstay in the treatment of infantile spasms in West syndrome, it has been shown that high-dose prednisolone at 8 mg/kg/day in divided doses for 2 weeks followed by rapid taper is very effective in abolishing spasms.[3] If the spasms do not disappear, ACTH can be initiated. The drug of choice for infantile spasms due to tuberous sclerosis is vigabatrin. Steroids and vigabatrin may also be combined.

It is important for the physician to be aware that some AEDs can actually worsen seizures, and can aggravate the problem. Absence seizures can worsen with CBZ and PHT. Myoclonic seizures can worsen with LTG, CBZ and PHT. CBZ and oxcarbamazepine may sometimes worsen seizures in benign rolandic epilepsy. Intravenous diazepam can sometimes precipitate tonic status epilepticus in Lennox-Gastaut syndrome.

When the clinical history is not clear as to whether a generalized tonic-clonic seizure is primarily generalized or which began focally before becoming generalized, it is better to initiate the patient on an AED which is effective for both focal as well as generalized seizures, the so-called broad-spectrum AED, e.g. are VPA, PB, ZNS and TPM.

The guidelines recommend the use of conventional AEDs (older AEDs) in most situations. Newer AEDs (second- and third-generation AEDs) are recommended when there is a contraindication to the use of older AEDs in certain coexisting illnesses, and when there is possibility of drug interaction, eg., when a person is on oral contraceptive pills, anticoagulants, antiretrovirals and immunosuppressive drugs.[4]

Steps in the Antiepileptic Drug Treatment

The first step in the management of newly diagnosed epilepsy is monotherapy—the use of a single AED. The response to first monotherapy in newly diagnosed epilepsy is excellent. Around 68% patients will become seizure-free at 1 year with monotherapy.[5] Around 47% of patients will respond to the first AED monotherapy.[6] Monotherapy also has fewer adverse effects.[7,8]

When the first monotherapy fails, one can take the second or the third steps in the management: one is to substitute the existing AED with another AED, a process called alternate monotherapy, or one can then choose to start a duotherapy.[9,10] The seizure freedom rate for the second and the third monotherapy trials is much lower, with only 14% becoming seizure-free for 1 year.[11] The efficacy of a second or a third AED monotherapy trial is much better if the reason for the failure of the first AED monotherapy was because of drug intolerance or an allergy, rather than because of lack of efficacy. Therefore, it is extremely important to choose the first AED carefully, taking into account the seizure type as well as the epilepsy syndrome. For example, if the seizure type is generalized tonic-clonic, and the epilepsy syndrome is an idiopathic generalized epilepsy such as juvenile myoclonic epilepsy, the drug of choice is VPA, while PHT and CBZ can worsen the condition.

Antiepileptic drug duotherapy or polytherapy: When one or two monotherapy trials fail, the next option is to combine two AEDs—a duotherapy trial. Combining two AEDs can have additive, supra-additive or antagonistic effects.[12] With the availability of more than 20 AEDs in the armamentarium, a large number of combinations is possible. Optimal combination of various AED is called "rational polytherapy"[13] which has been covered in detail in a separate Chapter.

When duotherapy fails: Despite the large number of newer AEDs with different mechanisms of action in the last two decades, nearly 25–30% of patients do not achieve seizure freedom, a figure that has remained so from the days of the first-generation AEDs.[4] When duotherapy fails, we can consider adding a third AED. The chances of achieving seizure freedom with addition of more than two AEDs are low, but are still worth trying as some 15–20% of those patients who failed many of the AEDs do achieve long-term remission with addition of one or other drug, be it older or newer AED.[14]

STEP 4: WHEN POLYTHERAPY FAILS

Around 20% of patients will be drug-resistant despite multiple trails of polytherapy. Around 50% of these patients are potential candidates for epilepsy surgery. Such patients are best referred to a comprehensive epilepsy unit which has the technical expertise to work up these patients for surgical candidacy.

Antiepileptic Drug Usage in Special Conditions

Antiepileptic drug choice in transplant patients: Enzyme-inducing drugs such as PHT, PB and CBZ reduce the levels of immunosuppressants like tacrolimus, sirolimus, cyclosporine and steroids. These drugs should be avoided. The most appropriate drugs that can be used after a liver transplantation are gabapentin, LEV and TPM. Following renal transplant, LTG, benzodiazepines and valproate are appropriate choices. Following bone marrow transplantation, gabapentin, LEV, LTG and TPM are safe.[15]

Antiepileptic drug choice in brain tumor patients: There is no role for AED prophylaxis in patients with brain tumor. Enzyme-inducing AEDs such as PHT, PB and CBZ must be avoided. These drugs may affect other treatment options like chemotherapy by enzyme induction. The most effective agents are LEV and valproate. Lamotrigine, LCM and gabapentin are also good choices.[15]

CONCLUSION

- There are three generations of AEDs, both older and newer, giving the physician a wide choice.
- Older AEDs (first-generation) are efficacious and inexpensive, but have more adverse effects, and pharmacokinetic and pharmacodynamic interactions.
- Newer AEDs (second-and third-generation) are expensive, but have fewer adverse effects, better tolerability and lesser pharmacokinetic and pharmacodynamic interactions.
- Choosing the right AED depends on several factors and must take into account the seizure type, epilepsy syndrome, gender, cost and associated comorbidities.
- Always start with monotherapy.
- Duotherapy must be chosen rationally, taking into consideration the mechanism of action of the AEDs.
- When the seizure type is not clear from history, choose an AED which is effective for both focal as well as generalized seizures.
- Some AEDs can aggravate seizures.

REFERENCES

1. Brodie MJ. Monostars: an aid to choosing an antiepileptic drug as monotherapy. Epilepsia. 1999;40 Suppl 6:S17-22.
2. Indian Epilepsy Society. (2008) Indian guidelines for the management of epilepsy: GEMIND. [online] Available from http://www.epilepsyindia.org/gemind-main.asp [Last accessed June, 2019].
3. Lux AL, Edwards SW, Hancock E, et al. The United Kingdom Infantile Spasms Study comparing vigabatrin with prednisolone or tetracosactide at 14 days: a multicentre, randomised controlled trial. Lancet. 2004;364:1773-8.
4. Johannessen SI, Landmark CJ. Antiepileptic drug interactions—principles and clinical implications. Curr Neuropharmacol. 2010;8:254-67.
5. Brodie MJ, Barry SJ, Bamagous GA, et al. Patterns of treatment response in newly diagnosed epilepsy. Neurology. 2012;78:1548-54.

6. Kwan P, Brodie MJ. Early identification of refractory epilepsy. N Engl J Med. 2000;342:314-9.
7. Reynolds EH, Shorvon SD. Monotherapy or polytherapy for epilepsy? Epilepsia. 1981;22:1-10.
8. Shorvon SD, Chadwick D, Galbraith AW, et al. One drug for epilepsy. Br Med J. 1978;1:474-6.
9. Beghi E, Gatti G, Tonini C, et al. Adjunctive therapy versus alternative monotherapy in patients with partial epilepsy failing on a single drug: a multicentre, randomised, pragmatic controlled trial. Epilepsy Res. 2003;57:1-13.
10. Kwan P, Brodie MJ. Epilepsy after the first drug fails: substitution or add-on? Seizure. 2000;9:464-8.
11. Mohanraj R, Brodie MJ. Diagnosing refractory epilepsy: response to sequential treatment schedules. Eur J Neurol. 2006;13:277-82.
12. Kwan P, Brodie MJ. Combination therapy in epilepsy: when and what to use. Drugs. 2006;66:1817-29.
13. French JA, Faught E. Rational polytherapy. Epilepsia. 2009;50 Suppl 8:63-8.
14. Callaghan BC, Anand K, Hesdorffer D, et al. Likelihood of seizure remission in an adult population with refractory epilepsy. Ann Neurol. 2007;62:382-9.
15. Ruiz-Giménez J, Sánchez-Alvarez JC, Cañadillas-Hidalgo F, et al. Antiepileptic treatment in patients with epilepsy and other comorbidities. Seizure. 2010;19:375-82.

11
CHAPTER

Rational Combination of Antiepileptic Drugs in the Management of Epilepsy

Sita Jayalakshmi, Suresh Babu Pasangulapati, Sudhindra Vooturi

INTRODUCTION

Over the past two decades, many antiepileptic drugs (AEDs) such as, felbamate, gabapentin, lacosamide, lamotrigine, levetiracetam, tiagabine, topiramate, oxcarbazepine, pregabalin, rufinamide, zonisamide, brivaracetam and perampanal have been approved by the Food and Drug Administration (FDA) based on results from formidable trials. While several of these second- and third-generation AEDs have proven monotherapy usage, most often they are indicated for adjunctive treatment of partial onset seizures, and thus leading to clinical use in polytherapy. Appropriate indications for AED polytherapy are—(1) transitional phase during titration of a new AED toward monotherapy; (2) transitional phase during titration of new AED for a relapse in epilepsy after considerable period of seizure control; and (3) in medically refractory epilepsy for long-term polytherapy. The concept of "rational polytherapy" is logical. Since persons with epilepsy (PWE) may either exhibit excessive neuronal excitation mediated by pro-glutamatergic influences or a failure of inhibition due to decreased GABAergic activity. Therefore, AED combinations when targeted over exuberant excitation and insufficient inhibition may perhaps be expected to be more efficient in seizure control.

An ever evolving armamentarium of AEDs offers both improved safety and tolerability. This advantage of new AEDs over older first-generation AEDs is a win-win situation both for the person with epilepsy and treating physician. This chapter considers an evidence-based practical approach for rational polytherapy in epilepsy.

NECESSITY FOR ANTIEPILEPTIC DRUG POLYTHERAPY

Long-term outcome studies often classify patients with newly diagnosed epilepsy into two distinct populations—easy to control and difficult to control.[1] Although more than 60% of patients become seizure free on first or second choice moderate doses of AEDs, the remaining one-third have pharmacoresistant epilepsy. A majority of these patients with medically intractable epilepsy often have an underlying structural cerebral abnormality.[2] Importantly, uncontrolled epilepsy is associated with excess mortality, cognitive and behavioral dysfunction.[3]

Kwan and Brodie reported that seizure control by first line/initial AED monotherapy is achieved in approximately two-thirds of PWE[1]. The remaining one-third are considered medically refractory; they are potential candidates for polytherapy, epilepsy surgery, or vagus nerve stimulation (VNS). The American Academy of Neurology/American Epilepsy Society (AAN/AES) Practice Guidelines for the treatment of refractory epilepsy recommends the use of second-generation AEDs for adjunctive treatment of refractory partial-onset seizures in adults.[4] While evidence from literature suggests that lamotrigine, oxcarbazepine and topiramate demonstrate overlapping efficacy; "no" ideal combination of AEDs has been identified. This is because of limitations to compare between trials due differences in patient demographics, seizure frequency, study design, blinding and inclusion/exclusion criteria.[4-6]

ANTIEPILEPTIC DRUG POLYTHERAPY—CURRENT EVIDENCE

Randomized AED polytherapy trials have reported that between 15% and 35% of patients with partial seizures become seizure free; additionally, up to 29% or more have a >50% seizure reduction.[7-9] One such trial, the Veteran Affairs I Cooperative Trial, a prospective, randomized trial, reported that 40% of patients who fails to achieve seizure control by phenytoin or carbamazepine monotherapy respond to polytherapy, with 11% of these patients becoming seizure free.[10]

WHAT IS RATIONAL POLYTHERAPY?

Rational polytherapy refers to the intentional choice of the second AED to enhance seizure control. It also presupposes that two AEDs with different mechanisms of action may provide better seizure control than two drugs with a similar mechanism. Anecdotally, it was believed that AED combinations with differing mechanisms of action will be more effective in seizure control than combinations with similar mechanisms of action.[11-13] However, polytherapy will not only produce additive, antagonistic, or synergistic efficacy in seizure control, but can also cause toxicity.[14] For example, combination of AEDs with competitive hepatic enzymatic metabolism or protein binding capacity not only produces antagonism in efficacy of one or both AEDs but also may lead to heightened toxicity. Importantly, AEDs with similar toxicity profiles could produce synergistic toxic effects.

Being aware of the various mechanisms of action of AEDs listed in the Table 1 below will help the physician to combine AEDs in optimizing polytherapy.

For a better understanding, AEDs are classified into two groups—(1) narrow spectrum drugs and (2) broad spectrum drugs.

1. Narrow-spectrum drugs are effective in partial seizures (with or without secondary generalization) and less effective in primarily generalized tonic-clonic seizures. In addition, these AEDs often worsen absence or myoclonic seizures.
2. Broad spectrum AEDs have good efficacy in partial and generalized seizures, and are especially useful in patients where the seizure type or the epilepsy syndrome is not characterized.

This classification though simplifies the understanding; plenty of research is required to comprehensively decode the mechanism of action of all AEDs. The list of narrow and broad spectrum AEDs is given in Table 2.

TABLE 1: Mechanism of action of antiepileptic drugs (AEDs).[15]

Antiepileptic drug	Mechanism of action
Sodium channel blockers	• Fast-inactivated state—phenytoin, carbamazepine, lamotrigine, oxcarbazepine, eslicarbazepine
	• Slow-inactivated state—lacosamide
Calcium channel blockers	• Low voltage activated channel—ethosuximide
	• High voltage activated channel—gabapentin, pregabalin
GABAergic drugs	• Prolongs chloride channel opening—barbiturates
	• Increased frequency of chloride channel opening—benzodiazepines
	• Inhibits GABA-transaminase—vigabatrin
	• Blocks synaptic GABA reuptake—tiagabine
Synaptic vesicle protein 2A modulation	• Levetiracetam
Carbonic anhydrase inhibition	• Acetazolamide
Multiple pharmacological targets	• Sodium valproate, felbamate, topiramate, zonisamide, rufinamide

Source: Brodie MJ, Sills GJ. Combining antiepileptic drugs—rational polytherapy? Seizure. 2011;20(5):369-75.

TABLE 2: **Broad and narrow spectrum antiepileptic drugs (AEDs).**

Broad spectrum AEDs	Narrow spectrum AEDs
• Sodium valproate	• Oxcarbazepine
• Clobazam	• Pregabalin
• Lamotrigine	• Lacosamide
• Topiramate	• Eslicarbazepine
• Levetiracetam	• Carbamazepine
• Zonisamide	• Phenytoin
• Rufinamide	• Ethosuximide

TABLE 3: **Polytherapy combinations based on mechanism of action.**

Polytherapy combination	Effect of polytherapy
• Sodium channel blocking AEDs + AEDs with GABA activity	• Synergistic action
• Sodium channel blocking AEDs + Broad spectrum AEDs	• Improved efficacy and tolerability
• Combination of two GABA mimetic drugs or AMPA and NMDA antagonists	• Improves efficacy but reduces tolerability
• Combination of two sodium channel blocking AEDs	• Reduces tolerability (not preferable)

(AEDs: antiepileptic drugs; AMPA: α-amino-3-hydroxy-5-methyl-4-isoxazolepropionic acid; GABA: gamma-aminobutyric acid; NMDA: N-methyl-D-aspartate)

Efficacy of AED polytherapy is particularly helpful in patients with multiple-seizure types where differing pharmacological properties improve efficacy. Similarly, patients with a single-seizure type may respond to a polytherapy that influences an individual ion channel or neurotransmitter system in different ways when AEDs with different mechanism of action are combined. Few effective AED polytherapy combinations based on mechanism of action are listed in Table 3.

Few AEDs with reported synergistic efficacy include—phenytoin and phenobarbital;[16] topiramate with carbamazepine, felbamate, lamotrigine, phenobarbital, or tiagabine;[14] valproate with phenytoin, carbamazepine, or ethosuximide[4,14] and levetiracetam.[6] Similarly, few other polytherapy combinations recommended include—sodium valproate with ethosuximide for absence seizures, sodium valproate with lamotrigine for partial-onset and generalized seizures and lamotrigine with topiramate for a range of seizure types.

Limited literature, retrospective case series report evidence favors a combination of sodium channel blocking AEDs with gamma-aminobutyric acid (GABA) activity.[17] Whereas, combining two GABA mimetic drugs or alpha-amino-3-hydroxy-5-methyl-4-isoxazolepropionicacid (AMPA) and N-methyl-D-aspartic acid (NMDA) antagonists although enhance efficacy but reduce tolerability.[17] Brodie et al.[18], in 105 patients receiving monotherapy with one of four AEDs (carbamazepine, phenobarbital, phenytoin, or valproate), reported that combination polytherapy with valproate and lamotrigine was more effective than any other combination (valproate-lamotrigine subgroup 64% responders, carbamazepine-lamotrigine 41% responders, phenytoin 38% responders). In a nutshell, a successful polytherapy includes cotherapies that (1) lack drug-drug interactions, (2) have a limited potential for amplification of adverse effects, and (3) reduce total drug load to achieve seizure control. Table 4 lists the proposed pharmacological targets of commonly used AEDs.[19]

POLYTHERAPY IN CLINICAL SETTING

Polytherapy is not proven in persons with new-onset epilepsy. Therefore, it is important that polytherapy is suggested in persons with failure to have seizure control after a well-tolerated, optimally administered monotherapy in an epilepsy syndrome that has been correctly diagnosed, often suggests of medically refractory epilepsy.[20] However, in persons with refractory epilepsy, "early" nonpharmacological treatments including epilepsy surgery should be strongly considered. Epilepsy surgery in suitable persons has been associated with improved quality of life, and reduced cost of treatment than chronic polytherapy.[21-24] Importantly, polytherapy increases the risk of teratogenesis in women with epilepsy of child bearing potential.[25-27]

Polytherapy, though indicated for medically refractory epilepsy, may have two different goals and courses; it may be transitional polytherapy (conversion to a second-line monotherapy) or chronic maintenance polytherapy to optimize seizure control and minimize adverse effects.

INITIATING ANTIEPILEPTIC DRUG POLYTHERAPY—LOOK BEFORE YOU LEAP

Polytherapy, though modestly improves efficacy, is always associated with increase in adverse effects. Therefore, before contemplating polytherapy, all patients should receive "at least" two sequential trials of optimal AED monotherapy using AEDs with differing mechanisms of action.

It is sensible to first evaluate the causes for failure of monotherapy before initiation of polytherapy. Few attributable causes for failure of monotherapy include:

- Nonepileptic seizures
- The patient has a combination of genuine epileptic and nonepileptic seizures

TABLE 4: The proposed pharmacological targets of commonly used antiepileptic drugs (AEDs).[18]

Drug	Sodium channels	Calcium channels/ currents	GABA receptors	GABA synapse	Glutamate receptor	Other
Older AEDs						
Benzodiazepines			+++			Abuse potential may limit use
Carbamazepine	+++	+	+			Modulates brain adenosine
Phenobarbital/ primidone			+++			Abuse potential may limit use
Ethosuximide		+++ (Modulates T-type currents)				Inhibits NADPH-linked aldehyde reductase (nesessary for gamma-hydroxybutyrate (GHB) synthesis; GHB can induce absences
Phenytoin	+++					
Valproate	+++	+ (Modulates T-types currents)		+		
Newer AEDs						
Felbamate	++	++		++	++	Idiosyncratic toxicity limits are
Gabapentin	+	++		+		
Lacosamide						Binds CRMP-2 receptor

(Continued)

(Continued)

Drug	Sodium channels	Calcium channels/ currents	GABA receptors	GABA synapse	Glutamate receptor	Other
Lamotrigine	+++	+				
Levetiracetam						Modulates presynaptic neurotransmitter release by SV2A receptor binding
Oxcarbazepine	+++	+				
Pregabalin		++				
Rufinamide	++					+?
Tiagabine				+++		
Topiramate	++	++	++	+	++	+ weak carbonic anhydrase inhibition
Zonisamide	+++	++ (Modulates T-type Currents)				++ facilities catecho laminergic and dopaminergic neurotransmission; + weak carbonic anhydrase inhibition

(+++: primary target; ++: probable target; +: possible target)

Source: St Louis EK. Truly "rational" polytherapy: maximizing efficacy and minimizing drug interactions, drug load and adverse effects. Curr Neuropharmacol. 2009;7(2):96-105.

- *Pseudo refractory epilepsy:* AED selected as monotherapy was not effective for the particular type of seizures. For example: a case of idiopathic generalized epilepsy being treated with phenytoin/carbamazepine
- Noncompliance to medications
- Precipitating factors for seizures (alcohol, sleep deprivation, stress).

The AED chosen for initial monotherapy should be based upon the seizure type (Table 5) and at an optimal dose (Table 6).

After eliminating the above mentioned causes for failure of monotherapy, additional investigations must be done to confirm if the epilepsy syndrome has been diagnosed aptly. Additional investigations also help in differential diagnosis by excluding alternative diagnosis and conditions that mimic epilepsy, for example psychogenic nonepileptic spells.[22,23] Ensuring correct diagnosis often avoids "unnecessary" polytherapy and its associated adverse effects.[24,25]

When initiating polytherapy, knowledge about potential pharmacokinetic and pharmacodynamics interactions is mandatory to avoid adverse events. The following are the pharmacokinetic interactions to consider:

- Potential cytochrome P450 (CYP) metabolism competition
- High percentage of protein binding.

TABLE 5: Recommended choice of antiepileptic drugs (AEDs) according to seizure type[19].

	Partial	Tonic-clonic	Absence	Myoclonic	Atonic/tonic
Phenobarbital	+	+	0	?+	?
Phenytoin	+	+	–	–	0
Carbamazepine	+	+	–	–	0
Sodium valporate	+	+	+	+	+
Ethosuximide	0	0	+	0	0
Benzodiazepines	+	+	?	+	+
Gabapentin	+	+	–	–	0
Lamotrigine	+	+	+	+	+
Oxcarbazepine	+	+	0	0	0
Topiramate	+	+	?	+	+
Tiagabine	+	+	–	–	0
Zonisamide	+	+	?+	+	?+
Levetiracetam	+	+	+	+	?
Felbamate	+	+	?+	?+	+
Vigabtrin	+	+	–	–	?

(+: efficacy; ?+: probable efficacy; 0: ineffective; –: worsens seizures; ?: unknown)

Source: St Louis EK. Truly "rational" polytherapy: maximizing efficacy and minimizing drug interactions, drug load and adverse effects. Curr Neuropharmacol. 2009;7(2):96-105.

TABLE 6: The optimal dosage of antiepileptic drugs (AEDs) as recommended by World Health Organization.[18]

Antiepileptic drug	Defined daily doses (mg)
Carbamazepine	1,000
Clonazepam	8
Phenobarbital	100
Phenytoin	300
Valproate	1,500
Oxcarbazepine	1,000
Lamotrigine	300
Topiramate	300
Zonisamide	200
Vigabatrin	2,000
Levetiracetam	1,500

Co-administration of enzyme-inducing AEDs [1,53](EIAEDs) (i.e. phenobarbital, phenytoin, or carbamazepine) with inducible AEDs (such as lamotrigine, oxcarbazepine, tiagabine, topiramate, or zonisamide). This coadministration often hastens metabolism of inducible AEDs, thus reducing drug concentrations and efficacy. On the contrary, when valproate, (an inhibitor of lamotrigine glucuronidation and clearance) is given with lamotrigine, there is a greater chance of serious rash than when lamotrigine is given in combination with EIAEDs.[28]

INITIATING ANTIEPILEPTIC DRUG POLYTHERAPY—CHOOSING THE RIGHT COMBINATION OF DRUGS

Two types of drug titration strategies have been often reported by randomized controlled trials.[29, 30.]

1. *Flexible dose titration*: Baseline AED dosage is reduced as needed to permit titration of adjunctive drug.
2. *Fixed dose titration*: Baseline AED dose is kept constant and the new AED is reduced to lower target dose.

Flexible dose titration approach was reportedly superior to fixed dose titration when evaluated for minimizing adverse effects especially that emerge during titration of a new adjunctive therapy. Unfortunately, there is no conclusive evidence to recommend a strategy to initiate third AED. However, while initiating a third AED, while maintaining the baseline AED regimens, titrating the third AED to a target dose and subsequently tapering off the least effective AED looks clinically reasonable. Sparse literature from recent studies suggest that two or three AEDs may effectively control seizures, however, four or more AEDs were not beneficial.[31] Importantly,

TABLE 7: Desirable and undesirable antiepileptic drug (AED) combinations.[18]

AED combination	Rationale	Desirability
Phenytoin (PHT) or carbamazepine (CBZ) plus		
Lamotrigine (LTG)	↓LTG and high adverse effects	No
Oxcarbazepine (OXC)	↓OXC and ↑PHT	No
Topiramate (TPM)	↓TPM and ↑PHT	No
Levetiracetam (LEV)	Possible synergism with CBZ	Yes
LTG or OXC plus		
Gabapentin (GBP)	Possible synergism	Yes
Pregabalin (PGB)	Possible synergism	Yes
LEV	Possible synergism	Yes
TPM	Possible synergism	Yes
Zonisamide (ZNS)	Possible additive	Yes/No
Valproate plus		
CBZ	↑CBZ epoxide	No
LTG	Evidence for efficacy and risk of rash	Yes/No
TPM	↑adverse effects	Yes/No
LEV	Possible synergism	Yes
ZNS	Possible synergism	Yes

Source: Brodie MJ, Yuen AW. Lamotrigine substitution study: evidence for synergism with sodium valproate? 105 Study Group. Epilepsy Res. 1997;26(3):423-32.

the same study reported that "inappropriate choice of second AED can lead to lack of efficacy in achieving seizure control, worsening of seizures, and increased side-effects".

Examples of some desirable AED combinations and undesirable combinations are shown in Table 7.

It is important to observe for adverse effect(s) that may develop during titration of the newest AED. Similar to adverse events, it is also important to opt an AED or polytherapy based on existing comorbidities of the patients (Table 8). Comorbid conditions may be physical, neuropsychological or psychiatric.

PHARMACOKINETICS

The newer AEDs have an advantage over the older AEDs because of their favorable pharmacokinetic and drug-drug interaction profiles. The older AEDs namely phenytoin, carbamazepine, phenobarbital and primidone have significant drug-drug interactions and are inducers of the CYP system (Fig. 1). The newer AEDs have better pharmacokinetics, with good oral bioavailability, low protein binding, linear kinetics, lack of active metabolites and low potential for drug-drug interactions.

TABLE 8: Choice of antiepileptic drug based on associated comorbidity.

Comorbidity	Recommended AED	AED to avoid
Headache	• Divalproate, Topiramate	
Anxiety, depression, psychosis, mood disorders	• Carbamazepine • Oxcarbazepine • Lamotrigine • Valproate	• Levetiracetam • Topiramate • Phenobarbitone
Sleep disturbances	• Clobazam	• Felbamate
Cognitive impairment	• Carbamazepine • Lamotrigine • Levetiracetam	• Topiramate • Phenobarbitone
Cardiac arrhythmias	• Valproate • Carbamazepine • Oxcarbazepine • Levetiracetam	• Lacosamide • Phenytoin • Rufinamide
Obesity	• Topiramate • Zonisamide	• Valproate
Attention Deficit disorder	• Valproate • Carbamazepine • Oxcarbazepine • Lamotrigine	• Phenobarbital • Benzodiazepines • Vigabatrin

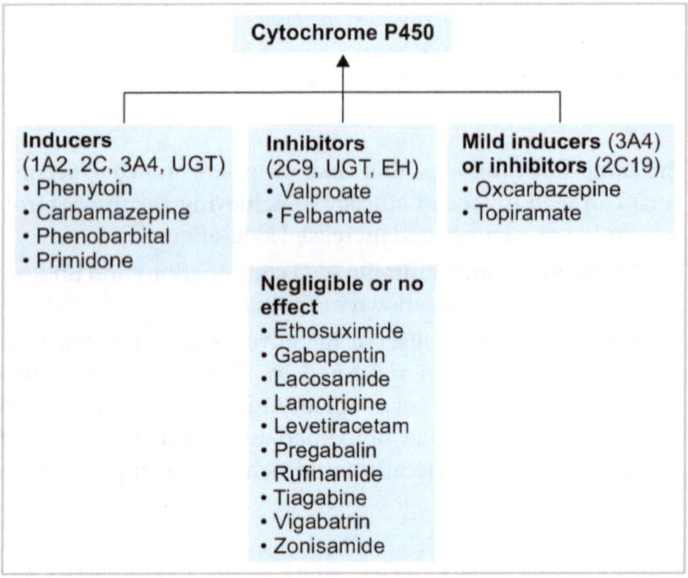

FIG. 1: Effects of antiepileptic drugs on the cytochrome P450.[32]

Source: Asconape JJ. The selection of antiepileptic drugs for the treatment of epilepsy in children and adults. Neurol Clin. 2010;28(4):843-52.

PHARMCOECONOMICS

In developing countries like India, affordability of medication is often associated with compliance to medication. With an

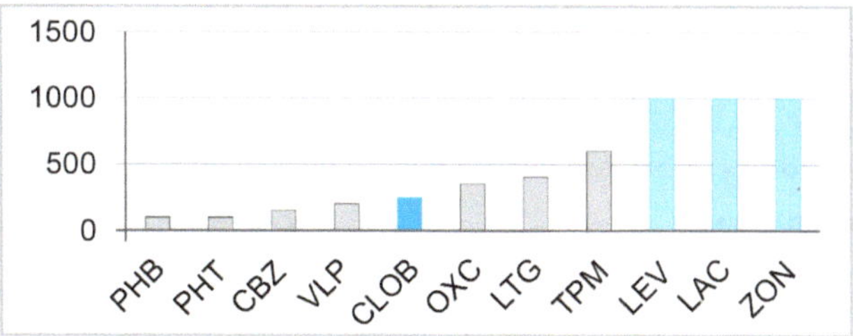

(PHB: phenobarbital; PHT: phenytoin; CBZ: carbamazepine; VLP: ventricular late potentials; CLOB: clobazam; OXC: oxcarbazepine; LTG: lamotrigine; TPM: topiramate; LEV: levetiracetam; LAC: lacosamide; ZON: zonisamide)

FIG. 2: Approximate cost of antiepileptic drug (AED) per month in rupees.

TABLE 9: Suggested combinations of antiepileptic drugs (AEDs).

Suggested combination	Example
• AEDs with different mechanisms of action	• A sodium channel blocker (lacosamide, lamotrigine) with nonsodium channel blockers (valproate, levetiracetam)
• Use AEDs combination with data of better efficacy in RCTS	• Carbamazepine with levetiracetam in partial epilepsy
• Use AEDs with favorable pharmacokinetic interactions	• Levetiracetam, lamotrigine and lacosamide
• Avoid combinations with similar mechanisms of action and/or unhelpful pharmacokinetic interactions	• Carbamazepine and phenytoin • Carbamazepine and lamotrigine

(RCTS: randomized controlled trials)

average per capita income of INR 3,685 in urban population and INR 1,360 in rural population, consider patient affordability while choosing an AED, especially the second AED is important because most of patients with epilepsy are often on prescribed medications for lifetime. The graph below gives an indication of the approximate expenses per month in rupees (y-axis) (Fig. 2).

PRESCRIBING ANTIEPILEPTIC DRUG POLYTHERAPY—WHICH DRUGS TO COMBINE?

Combination of AEDs with differing mechanisms of action is superior to combinations of AEDs with similar cellular effects. Early trials in drug laboratories suggest a combination of a single mechanism drug with an AED known to possess multiple mechanisms of action as most successful. Table 9 and Table 10 summarize the suggested combinations and rationale for the same.

TABLE 10: Mechanisms for common antiepileptic drugs (AED) interactions.[18]

Combination	Desirability	Rationale
Pheytoin or carbamazepine, plus		
Lamotrigine	–	EIAEDs decrease LTG, heightened pharmacodyramic neurotoxic adverse effects
Oxcarbazepine	–	EIAEDs decrease OXC, OXC inhibits CYP2C19 and may increase PHT concentrations; increased neurotoxic asverese effects
Topiramate	–	EIAEDs decrease TPM, TPM inhibits CYP2C19 and may increase PHT concentrations; increased neurotoxic adverse effects
Levetiracetam	+	Posssible synergism with CBZ
Lamotrigine or oxcarbazepine, plus		
Gabapentin	++	Potential synergism
Pregabalin	++	Potential synergism
Levetiracetam	++	Potential synergism
Topiramate	+	Potential synergism
Zonisamide	+/–	Possible additive effects, similar principle MOA
Valproate or divalproex, plus		
Phenytoin	–	Increased free PHT fraction and neurotoxic adverse effects, however, retrospective case series suggest synergism
Carbamazepine	–	Valporate increases CBZ-epoxide, similar principle MOA
Lamotrigine	+/–	Controlled clinical trial evidence for efficacy; however, increased risk of rash
Topiramate	+/–	Hypothetically may offset weight gain adverse effects; however, increase in neurotoxic adverse effects
Levetiracetam	++	Possible synergism
Zonisamide	+	Possible synergism

(+: potentially desirable combination; ++: desirable combiantion; –:potentially undesirable combination; – :undesirable combination; +/–: data are confliciting)

Source: Brodie MJ, Yuen AW. Lamotrigine substitution study: evidence for synergism with sodium valproate? 105 Study Group. Epilepsy Res. 1997;26(3):423-32.

POTENTIAL ADVERSE EFFECTS OF POLYTHERAPY

Commonly reported adverse effects of AED polytherapy include dose-related neurotoxic and cognitive side effects.[33,34]

Cognitive impairments are commonly reported only when specifically questioning the patient. Therefore, periodic detailed neuropsychological and electrophysiological measures should be done to assess impairments in attention, concentration, executive function and memory in patients receiving AED therapy.[35-40] Additionally, routine use of AED specific adverse event screening instruments during office visits may help early identification of patients with adverse effects that limit quality of life.[34,35] For example, AED like topiramate have a higher incidence of pharmacodynamics adverse effects when used as an adjunctive in polytherapy as when it is administered as monotherapy.[30,40-42]

CHOOSE POLYTHERAPY NOT OVERTREATMENT

Overtreatment is often defined as an excessive polytherapy with "suboptimal" risk-to-benefit ratio.[33,43] It is important to note that both uncontrolled seizures and polytherapy are independently associated with decreased quality of life in PWE.[75] Paradoxically, reduction in polytherapy can lead to improved seizure control in two-thirds of patients.[33,43] Therefore, judicious use of polytherapy is advocated and considering reducing polytherapy can result in reduced risk of serious adverse effects by minimizing drug interactions,[12] and also decreasing costs.[22] It has to be remembered that polytherapy is less tolerable than monotherapy due to higher total drug load, which is the sum of the prescribed daily doses (PDD) of AEDs.[44,45] To avoid neurological side-effects, the ratio of the PDD and the average effective or defined daily dose (DDD) should not exceed 2.[44,46,47] It is important to note that monotherapy or polytherapy in comparable drug loads show no difference in perceived adverse effects. Therefore, in clinical practice; when the addition of another AED is required, PDD/DDD ratio should be used to calculate the total dose a patient would tolerate.

DRAWBACKS OF ANTIEPILEPTIC DRUG POLYTHERAPY

The three major problems of AED polytherapy are chronic toxicity, unfavorable interactions and difficulty in evaluating individual pharmacological effects.

Polytherapy is associated with decreased patient compliance, lower quality of life, and higher costs. In fact, polytherapy is a predictive factor for reduced bone mineral density.[48] Therefore, polytherapy should be exclusively reserved for patients where options like epilepsy surgery and/or vagal nerve stimulation are not feasible. However, breakthrough seizures are a potential possibility while reducing polytherapy. Encouragingly, epilepsy surgery has been shown to successfully eliminate the necessity for polytherapy especially after successful anterior temporal lobectomy.[49-51] Moreover, adjunctive VNS therapy as an adjunct has been shown to decrease total drug load by reducing the total number of AEDs and/or decreased doses of individual AEDs.[47]

CONCLUSION

Monotherapy is always preferred over polytherapy in PWE. However, polytherapy may help a substantial number of patients with medically refractory epilepsy. Polytherapy should be considered during conversion to a new monotherapy, especially in relapse of epilepsy and for chronic maintenance in people with refractory epilepsy. Importantly, polytherapy should be continued only when improved efficacy outweighs adverse effects. Avoiding overtreatment will result in reducing adverse effects, drug interactions and cost.

REFERENCES

1. Kwan P, Brodie MJ. Early identification of refractory epilepsy. N Engl J Med 2000;342(5):314-9.
2. Dlugos DJ, Sammel MD, Strom BL, et al. Response to first drug trial predicts outcome in childhood temporal lobe epilepsy. Neurology. 2001;57(12): 2259-64.
3. Sillanpää M, Jalava M, Kaleva O, et al. Long-term prognosis of seizures with onset in childhood. N Engl J Med. 1998;338(24):1715-22.
4. Cramer JA, Fisher R, Ben-Menachem E, et al. New antiepileptic drugs: comparison of key clinical trials. Epilepsia. 1999;40(5):590-600.
5. French JA, Kanner AM, Bautista J, et al. Efficacy and tolerability of the new antiepileptic drugs II: treatment of refractory epilepsy: report of the Therapeutics and Technology Assessment Subcommittee and Quality Standards Subcommittee of the American Academy of Neurology and the American Epilepsy Society. Neurology. 2004;62(8):1261-73.
6. Marson A, Beghi E, Berg A, et al. The Cochrane collaboration: systematic reviews and their relevance to epilepsy. The Cochrane Epilepsy Network. Epilepsia. 1996;37(10):917-921.
7. Crawford P, Chadwick D. A comparative study of progabide, valproate, and placebo as add-on therapy in patients with refractory epilepsy. J Neurol Neurosurg Psychiatry. 1986;49(11):1251-7.
8. Murri L, Iudice A. Vigabatrin as first add-on treatment in carbamazepine-resistant epilepsy patients. Acta Neurol Scand Suppl. 1995;162:40-2.
9. Tanganelli P, Regesta G. Vigabatrin vs. carbamazepine monotherapy in newly diagnosed focal epilepsy: a randomized response conditional cross-over study. Epilepsy Res. 1996;25(3):257-62.
10. Mattson RH, Cramer JA, Collins JF. A comparison of valproate with carbamazepine for the treatment of complex partial seizures and secondarily generalized tonic-clonic seizures in adults. The Department of Veterans Affairs Epilepsy Cooperative Study No. 264 Group. N Engl J Med. 1992;327(11):765-71.
11. Leppik IE. Monotherapy and polypharmacy. Neurology 2000;55(11 Suppl 3): S25-9.
12. Perucca E. Pharmacological principles as a basis for polytherapy. Acta Neurol Scand Suppl. 1995;162:31-4.

13. Schmidt D. Modern management of epilepsy: Rational polytherapy. Baillieres Clin Neurol. 1996;5(4):757-63.
14. Czuczwar SJ, Borowicz KK. Polytherapy in epilepsy: the experimental evidence. Epilepsy Res. 2002;52(1):15-23.
15. Brodie MJ, Sills GJ. Combining antiepileptic drugs--rational polytherapy? Seizure. 2011;20(5):369-75.
16. Bourgeois BF. Antiepileptic drug combinations and experimental background: the case of phenobarbital and phenytoin. Naunyn Schmiedebergs Arch Pharmacol. 1986;333(4):406-11.
17. Deckers CL, Czuczwar SJ, Hekster YA, et al. Selection of antiepileptic drug polytherapy based on mechanisms of action: the evidence reviewed. Epilepsia. 2000;41(11):1364-74.
18. Brodie MJ, Yuen AW. Lamotrigine substitution study: evidence for synergism with sodium valproate? 105 Study Group. Epilepsy Res. 1997;26(3):423-32.
19. St Louis EK. Truly "rational" polytherapy: maximizing efficacy and minimizing drug interactions, drug load and adverse effects. Curr Neuropharmacol. 2009;7(2): 96-105.
20. Kwan P, Brodie MJ. Effectiveness of first antiepileptic drug. Epilepsia. 2001;42(10)::1255-60.
21. Bien CG, Kurthen M, Baron K, et al. Long-term seizure outcome and antiepileptic drug treatment in surgically treated temporal lobe epilepsy patients: a controlled study. Epilepsia 2001;42(11):1416-21.
22. Boon P, D'Have M, Van Walleghem P, et al. Direct medical costs of refractory epilepsy incurred by three different treatment modalities: a prospective assessment. Epilepsia. 2002;43(1):96-102.
23. Kuzniecky R, Rubin ZK, Faught E, et al. Antiepileptic drug treatment after temporal lobe epilepsy surgery: a randomized study comparing carbamazepine and polytherapy. Epilepsia 1992;33(5):908-12.
24. Kwan P, Brodie MJ. Drug treatment of epilepsy: when does it fail and how to optimize its use? CNS Spectr. 2004;9(2):110-9.
25. Crawford P. Epilepsy and pregnancy. Seizure. 2002;11 Suppl. A:212-9.
26. Pennell PB. Antiepileptic drug pharmacokinetics during pregnancy and lactation. Neurology. 2003;61(6 Suppl 2):S35-42.
27. Oguni M, Osawa M. Epilepsy and pregnancy. Epilepsia. 2004;45 Suppl 8:37-41.
28. Arroyo S, de la Morena A. Life-threatening adverse events of antiepileptic drugs. Epilepsy Res. 2001;47(1-2):155-74.
29. St Louis EK, Gidal BE, Henry TR, et al. Conversions between monotherapies in epilepsy: expert consensus. Epilepsy Behav. 2007;11(2):222-34.
30. Naritoku DK, Hulihan JF, Schwarzman LK, et al. Effect of cotherapy reduction on tolerability of epilepsy add-on therapy: a randomized controlled trial. Ann Pharmacother 2005;39(3):418-23.
31. Stephen LJ, Brodie MJ. Seizure freedom with more than one antiepileptic drug. Seizure. 2002;11(6):349-51.
32. Asconape JJ. The selection of antiepileptic drugs for the treatment of epilepsy in children and adults. Neurol Clin. 2010;28(4):843-52.
33. Deckers CL. Overtreatment in adults with epilepsy. Epilepsy Res. 2002;52(1):43-52.
34. Gilliam FG, Fessler AJ, Baker G, et al. Systematic screening allows reduction of adverse antiepileptic drug effects: a randomized trial. Neurology. 2004;62(1):23-7.
35. Meador KJ, Loring DW, Moore EE, et al. Comparative cognitive effects of phenobarbital, phenytoin, and valproate in healthy adults. Neurology. 1995;45(8):1494-9.
36. Meador KJ. Cognitive outcomes and predictive factors in epilepsy. Neurology. 2002;58(8 Suppl 5):S21-6.
37. Rahmann A, Stodieck S, Husstedt IW, et al. Pre-attentive cognitive processing in epilepsy. A pilot study on the impact of epilepsy type and anti-epileptic treatment. Eur Neurol. 2002;48(3):146-52.
38. Trimble MR, Thompson PJ. Anticonvulsant drugs, cognitive function and behavior. Epilepsia. 1983;24 Suppl 1:S55-63.

39. Vining EP. Cognitive dysfunction associated with antiepileptic drug therapy. Epilepsia. 1987;28 Suppl 2:S18-22.
40. Nadkarni S, LaJoie J, Devinsky O. Current treatments of epilepsy. Neurology. 2005;64(12 Suppl 3):S2-11.
41. Privitera MD, Brodie MJ, Mattson RH, et al. Topiramate, carbamazepine and valproate monotherapy: double-blind comparison in newly diagnosed epilepsy. Acta Neurol Scand. 2003;107(3):165-75.
42. Reife R, Pledger G, Wu SC. Topiramate as add-on therapy: pooled analysis of randomized controlled trials in adults. Epilepsia. 2000;41 Suppl 1:S66-71.
43. Schmidt D, Elger C, Holmes GL. Pharmacological overtreatment in epilepsy: mechanisms and management. Epilepsy Res. 2002;52(1):3-14.
44. Deckers CL, Hekster YA, Keyser A, et al. Reappraisal of polytherapy in epilepsy: a critical review of drug load and adverse effects. Epilepsia. 1997;38(5):570-5.
45. Deckers CL, Hekster YA, Keyser A, et al. Monotherapy versus polytherapy for epilepsy: a multicenter double-blind randomized study. Epilepsia. 2001;42(11):1387-94.
46. Deckers CL, Genton P, Sills GJ, et al. Current limitations of antiepileptic drug therapy: a conference review. Epilepsy Res. 2003;53(1-2):1-17.
47. Labar DR. Antiepileptic drug use during the first 12 months of vagus nerve stimulation therapy: a registry study. Neurology. 2002;59(6 Suppl 4):S38-43.
48. El-Hajj Fuleihan G, Dib L, Yamout B, et al. Predictors of bone density in ambulatory patients on antiepileptic drugs. Bone. 2008;43(1):149-55.
49. Maher J, McLachlan RS. Antiepileptic drug treatment following temporal lobectomy. Neurology. 1998;51(1):305-7.
50. Schiller Y, Cascino GD, So EL, et al. Discontinuation of antiepileptic drugs after successful epilepsy surgery. Neurology. 2000;54(2):346-9.
51. Wieser HG, Hane A. Antiepileptic drug treatment before and after selective amygdalohippocampectomy. Epilepsy Res. 2003;55(3):211-23.

12
CHAPTER

Individualizing Treatment for Drug Monitoring Therapeutics

Shyam K Jaiswal

INTRODUCTION

There has been a significant shift in the treatment of epilepsy, from "one dose fits all patients" in the early days to individualised treatment of patient. Over the past 50 years, therapeutic drug monitoring (TDM) has helped in understanding pharmacological variability of antiepileptic drugs (AEDs). There are various factors that can contribute to pharmacokinetic variability that include physiological factors (gender, age and pregnancy), external factors (such as food and co-medication), pathological conditions (liver/kidney dysfunction) and genetic factors (polymorphisms in metabolising enzymes). Special attention is required for children, pregnant women and the elderly, in whom the most extensive pharmacokinetic changes occur. There are also challenges regarding the use and misuse of TDM, such as the use of drug monitoring without a clear indication, misinterpretation of the reference range, and erroneous sampling times.

Dosing Strategies-assessing Efficacy and Tolerability in Relation to Serum Concentration Measurements

Buchthal and co-workers were the first to publish studies on serum concentrations of phenytoin and phenobarbital and their relation to clinical effects,[1] findings inspiring further pharmacokinetic studies on AEDs.[2] This resulted in a series of books about AEDs starting with AEDs by Woodbury et al. (1972).[3] A series of workshops, known as Workshop on the Determination of Antiepileptic Drugs in Body Fluids (WODADIBOF), took place between 1972 and 1979[4] that established a multidisciplinary collaboration between pharmacologists, pharmacists, toxicologists, neurologists and paediatricians. It was anticipated that new information concerning the relationship of serum concentrations to seizure control and toxicity would improve utilisation of AEDs.

Many new AEDs have become available during the past 50 years, and the knowledge of variability between patients or within the same patients treated with one AED, or combinations of several AEDs, has evolved. New challenges in dosing of AEDs include the wide range of combinations of AEDs available, many possible pharmacokinetic drug interactions, and changes in pharmacokinetics due to physiological changes in various patient groups.

Terminology and Definitions

The International League Against Epilepsy (ILAE) position paper recommends the use of two different terms to define drug concentration ranges in relation to their clinical effects.[5]

A reference range is defined as a range of drug concentrations quoted by a laboratory with a lower limit for therapeutic response and an upper limit above which toxicity is more likely to occur.

A therapeutic range is defined as the range of drug concentrations associated with the optimal response in a certain patient and may vary between patients. This individual therapeutic concentration is considered a better guide to individualisation than reference ranges.[5]

Various Factors Affecting Pharmacokinetics

External Factors

External factors like environmental factors, such as cigarette smoking, food and drink can affect drug pharmacokinetics. Hepatic enzymes, such as phase I cytochrome P450 (CYP), more specifically CYP3A4, may be inhibited by intake of grapefruit juice. Smoking may induce certain CYPs (CYP1A2) and phase II uridine diphosphate-glucuronosyltransferases (UGTs) (UGT1A4). Comedication with AEDs have a pronounced potential to cause pharmacokinetic interactions, as there are both strong enzyme inhibitors (valproic acid, stiripentol and felbamate) and inducers (car-bamazepine, phenytoin and phenobarbital).

Physiological Factors and Concurrent Illness

Physiological changes such as pregnancy and elderly age can change pharmacokinetics. Comborbid illness, such as hepatic or renal failure affect drug metabolism significantly.

Genetic Factors

Another cause of pharmacokinetic variability is genetic polymorphisms in drug metabolising enzymes, which may be revealed by genotyping.[6-8] However, in many cases it is easier to monitor the serum concentration.

Nonadherence

Nonadherence is very common issue with any chronic illness. The use of TDM may reveal poor or variable adherence. By using TDM data, poor adherence has been shown to be a major reason for hospitalisation due to break-through seizures (when serum concentrations were <50% of baseline values), even in patients denying nonadherence.[9]

Implementation of Therapeutic Drug Monitoring

The TDM concept rests on the assumption that clinical effects correlate better with drug concentrations than with dose. TDM has become of value in the treatment of epilepsy since it is difficult to determine the optimal dose on clinical grounds alone as discussed above.[5,10] The aim of TDM is to adjust for pharmacokinetic variability to optimise drug therapy in the individual patient. Proposed indications for TDM of AEDs are summarised in Box 1 and pharmacokinetic characteristics of AEDs in Table 1. The process of therapeutic drug monitoring is discussed in Flowchart 1.

BOX 1 Therapeutic drug monitoring (TDM): Practical recommendations.

Various Indications of TDM Includes

- At AED initiation
- Dose changes, esepcially with nonlinear pharmacokinetics
- Special population (preganancy, elderly)
- Suspicion of toxicity or overdose
- Drug failure with suspicion of poor adeherence
- Change in formulations
- Co-morbidities like hepatic and renal failure
- In status epilepticus or emergency situations

TABLE 1: Reference range for antiepileptic drugs.

Drugs	Reference concentration range (mg/L)
Carbamazepine	4–12
Lacosamide	5–10
Lamotrigine	2.5–15
Levetiracetam	12–46
Perampanel	0.2–0.8
Phenobarbital	10–35
Phenytoin	10–20
Sodium Valproate	6–22
Topiramate	5–20
Zonisamide	10–40

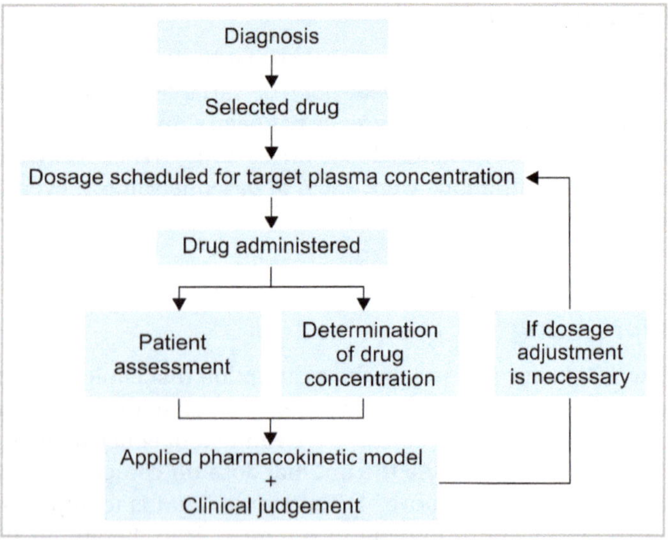

FLOWCHART 1: Process of therapeutic drug monitoring.

How to Measure TDM?

- Serum or plasma concentration
- Free/unbound concentration if very high protein binding (>90%) such as phenytoin and valproic acid
- Saliva sampling is being explored.

When to Take Blood Sample?

- For most AEDs, the total concentration of bound and unbound drug of the main active compound is measured.
- The blood sampling time should be standardised in the morning before intake of the dose at assumed steady state.[11]

Experience with the Recent and Most Recent Antiepileptic Drugs

Among the newer, second generation AEDs, the following may be good candidates for TDM felbamate, gabapentin, lamotrigine, levetiracetam, oxcarbazepine, pregabalin, tiagabine, topiramate and zonisamide, since these drugs show marked pharmacokinetic variability likely to contribute to differences in dosage requirements.[12,13] The most recently available AEDs include eslicarbazepine acetate, lacosamide, perampanel, rufinamide and stiripentol. Various studies demonstrate extensive pharmacokinetic variability and potential for interactions also for these drugs.[14-18]

For AEDs with short half-lives (levetiracetam, gabapentin, pregabalin and tiagabine), interpretation of TDM data may be complicated due to fluctuations in serum concentrations within the dosing interval, causing variability, if the blood sampling time is not well standardized.

Serum Concentrations of Metabolites

Some AEDs have pharmacological active metabolites. For instance, primidone is metabolised to phenylethylmalonamide and phenobarbital. Most often, the concentration of the derived phenobarbital is used. For drugs for which the parent molecule and active metabolite are present at high concentrations (i.e. clobazam and N-desmethylclobazam), both can be measured and various metabolite/parent compound ratios used in the interpretation of the results.[19]

Unbound Drug Concentrations

Measurement of the unbound drug concentration may be of importance in special situations, since this is the fraction of the drug that is pharmacologically active. In certain situations, the level of binding of a drug to plasma proteins may be lower than normal, in which case measuring the total concentration can be misleading and may lead to an underestimation of the amount of pharmacologically active drug. This is, however, only relevant when interpreting the serum concentrations of highly-protein-bound (>90%) drugs, such as phenytoin and valproic acid,[5] as well as some of the newer AEDs, i.e. tiagabine, stiripentol and perampanel.[12]

Saliva Concentrations and Blood Spots

Saliva is being explored as alternative medium for several AEDs,[20] since the concentration in saliva reflects the unbound concentration in serum. Saliva sampling is simple and noninvasive and is useful in children who fear venepuncture. The saliva concentrations may, however, be affected by the sampling conditions and contamination of mucus and the presence of residual drug and food.

The Future Dosing Strategies toward Improved Personalised Medicine

More studies are warranted in special patient populations regarding pharmacokinetic variability. This will contribute to better understanding of the need to individualise treatment with AEDs. Recent initiatives from the European Medicines Agency (EMA) now support further the implementation of pharmacogenomics in drug development and surveillance.[21] Genetically susceptible subgroups of patients can avoid certain drugs and hence possible toxic or fatal effects. Consequently, more tailored therapy might be offered to the individual patient in the future using a combination of TDM and pharmacogenomic test panels.[22]

Overuse of TDM?

Criticism has been directed toward the overuse of TDM and the method should obviously not be used without clear indications. It was stated that "treating patients is much more important than treating blood concentrations".[23]

There are also several pitfalls regarding the interpretation of TDM results. There is no strict correlation between efficacy and toxicity of an AED and the corresponding serum concentration in individual patients.[24] The establishment of individual therapeutic concentrations that differ from the suggested reference ranges may be challenging to accept for the clinician and the patient.

There is a lack of class I evidence of the clinical impact of TDM on treatment outcome in epilepsy. In a Cochrane review of TDM of AEDs in epilepsy patients from 2007, only one study met the inclusion criteria by assessing efficacy outcomes of AED monotherapy with or without TDM.[25] It was concluded that there was no clear evidence to support aiming at predefined target ranges,[26] which, however, no longer is recommended practice.[5] So far, there are no other studies in which the impact of implementation of TDM on outcome of epilepsy treatment has been investigated as a primary goal.

CONCLUSION

We have learned from history, and through application of TDM, that the use of AEDs implies variability regarding dose and serum concentration relationships, due to external, physiological, as well as genetic factors. Patient groups, such as children, pregnant women and the elderly, in whom the most extensive pharmacokinetic changes occur, need special attention and close follow-up of their treatment, as do patients with complicated and changing combination treatments. The main reasons for misuse of TDM include use of TDM without a clear indication, misinterpretation of the reference range, and erroneous sampling times. AED therapy should be tailored to the individual patient for an optimal treatment outcome and balance between efficacy and tolerability, and TDM can, in many situations, facilitate this strategy.

REFERENCES

1. Buchthal F, Svensmark O. Aspects of the pharmacology of phenytoin (Dilantin) and phenobarbital relevant to their dosage in the treatment of epilepsy. Epilepsia. 1960;1:373-84.
2. Kutt H, Wintes W, Kokenge R, et al. Diphenylhydantoin metabolism, blood levels, and toxicity. Arch Neurol. 1964;11:642-8.

3. Woodbury DM, Penry JK, Schmidt RP, eds. Antiepileptic Drugs. USA: Raven Press; 1972.
4. Meijer JWA, Meinardi H, Gardener-Thorpe C, et al. Methods of analysis of anti-epileptic drugs. Amsterdam: Excerpta Medica (New York: American Elsevier); 1973.
5. Patsalos PN, Berry DJ, Bourgeois BF, et al. Antiepileptic drugs—best practice guidelines for therapeutic drug monitoring: a position paper by the subcommission on therapeutic drug monitoring, ILAE Commission on Therapeutic Strategies. Epilepsia. 2008;49(7):1239-76.
6. Sirot JE, van der Velden JW, Rentsch K, et al. Therapeutic drug monitoring and pharmacogenetic tests as tools in pharmacovigilance. Drug Saf. 2006;29(9):735-68.
7. Löscher W, Klotz U, Zimprich F, et al. The clinical impact of pharmacogenetics on the treatment of epilepsy. Epilepsia. 2009;50(1):1-23.
8. Cascorbi I. The promises of personalized medicine. Eur J Clin Pharmacol. 2010;66(8): 749-54.
9. Samsonsen C, Reimers A, Bråthen G, et al. Nonadherence to treatment causing acute hospitalizations in people with epilepsy: an observational, prospective study. Epilepsia. 2014;55(11):e125-8.
10. Koch-Weser J. Serum drug concentrations in clinical perspective. Ther Drug Monit. 1981;3(1):3-16.
11. Tomson T, Johannessen SI. Therapeutic drug monitoring of new antiepileptic drugs. Eur J Clin Pharmacol. 2000;55(10):697-705.
12. Krasowski MD, McMillin GA. Advances in anti-epileptic drug testing. Clin Chim Acta. 2014;436:224-36.
13. Johannessen Landmark C, Johannessen SI, Tomson T. Host factors affecting antiepileptic drug delivery- Pharmacokinetic variability. Adv Drug Delivery Rev. 2012;64(10):896-910.
14. Perucca E, Cloyd J, Critchley D, et al. Rufinamide: clinical pharmacokinetics and concentration-response relationships in patients with epilepsy. Epilepsia. 2008;49(7):1123-41.
15. May TW, Boor R, Mayer T, et al. Concentrations of stiripentol in children and adults with epilepsy: the influence of dose, age, and comedication. Ther Drug Monit. 2012;34(4):390-7.
16. Markoula S, Teotonio R, Ratnaraj N, et al. Lacosamide serum concentrations in adult patients with epilepsy: the influence of gender, age, dose, and concomitant antiepileptic drugs. Ther Drug Monit. 2014;36(4):494-8.
17. Johannessen Landmark C, Svendsen T, Dinarevic J, et al. The impact of pharmacokinetic interactions with eslicarbazepine acetate versus oxcarbazepine and carbamazepine in clinical practice. Ther Drug Monit. 2016;38(4):499-505.
18. Patsalos PN, Gougoulaki M, Sander JW. Perampanel serum concentrations in adults with epilepsy: effect of dose, age, sex, and concomitant anti-epileptic drugs. Ther Drug Monit. 2016;38(3):358-64.
19. Burns ML, Baftiu A, Opdahl MS, et al. Therapeutic drug monitoring of clobazam and its metabolite—impact of age and comedication on pharmacokinetic variability. Ther Drug Monit 2016;38(3):350-7.
20. Patsalos PN, Berry DJ. Therapeutic drug monitoring of antiepileptic drugs by use of saliva. Ther Drug Monit. 2013;35(1):4-29.
21. Ehmann F, Caneva L, Papaluca M. European Medicines Agency initiatives and perspectives on pharmacogenomics. Br J Clin Pharmacol. 2014;77(4):612-7.
22. Hiemke C, Shams M. Phenotyping and genotyping of drug metabolism to guide pharmacotherapy in psychiatry. Curr Drug Deliv. 2013;10(1):46-53.
23. Chadwick DW. Overuse of monitoring of blood concentrations of antiepileptic drugs. Br Med J (Clin Res Ed) 1987;294(6574):723-4.
24. St Louis EK. Monitoring antiepileptic drugs: a level-headed approach. Curr Neuropharmacol. 2009;7(2):115-9.
25. Tomson T, Dahl ML, Kimland E. Therapeutic drug monitoring of antiepileptic drugs for epilepsy. Cochrane Database Syst Rev. 2007;(1):CD002216.
26. Januzzi G, Cian P, Fattore C, et al. A multicenter randomized controlled trial on the clinical impact of therapeutic drug monitoring in patients with newly diagnosed epilepsy. The Italian TDM study group. Epilepsia. 2000;41(2):222-30.

13
CHAPTER

Management of Status Epilepticus

Aniruddha Vasant More, Arun Garg

INTRODUCTION

Status epilepticus is a devastating and potentially life-threatening emergency commonly encountered in routine practice. It can lead to permanent brain damage or mortality if not treated timely and aggressively. Hence a physician should be familiar with management of status epilepticus when he encounters such a patient in his practice.

DEFINITION

Previously status epilepticus was defined as continuous seizure activity lasting for more than 30 minutes or if the patient has two or more seizures without regaining consciousness between seizures.[1] As per the International League Against Epilepsy (ILAE), status epilepticus is a condition resulting either from the failure of the mechanisms responsible for seizure termination or from the initiation of mechanisms, which lead to abnormally, prolonged seizures (after time point t1). It is a condition, which can have long-term consequences (after time point t2), including neuronal death, neuronal injury and alteration of neuronal networks, depending on the type and duration of seizures.[2]

So in this definition, two time periods are stated, t1 is the time after which seizure has tendency to become self-sustaining (unless intervened) and it can be considered as continuous seizure activity and t2 is the time after which ongoing seizure can cause permanent neuronal damage. T1 and t2 times for different seizures have been defined. For generalized tonic-clonic seizures, t1 is 5 minutes and t2 is 30 minutes while for focal seizures with impaired awareness t1 and t2 times are 10 minutes and 60 minutes, respectively. So for practical purpose any generalized convulsive tonic-clonic seizure lasting for more than 5 minutes should be considered as status epilepticus and prompt treatment should be started.

NONCONVULSIVE STATUS EPILEPTICUS

When the seizures have obvious motor manifestations, they are called as convulsions. However, if the seizure activity is going on in the brain as evidenced by electroencephalogram (EEG) record but no obvious motor manifestations are seen clinically then such seizures are called as nonconvulsive seizures. In comatose patients or patients with underlying encephalopathy who have unexplained altered sensorium without any apparent cause, if the total duration of seizure activity in the EEG is more than 30 minutes in any given hour of EEG record then it is called nonconvulsive status epilepticus (NCSE). Consensus EEG criteria have been developed for diagnosis of NCSE called as "Salzburg EEG criteria for NCSE".[3] NCSE is frequently encountered in the intensive care unit (ICU) setting. A high index of suspicion is necessary to diagnose NCSE and it should be suspected in patients who have unexplained altered sensorium. Subtle clinical stereotyped signs like nystagmus, gaze deviation, hippus, face and limb twitching, autonomic instability, chewing, episodic posturing of limbs may give a clue that patient is having an ongoing seizure.

REFRACTORY STATUS EPILEPTICUS

When seizure continues despite giving adequate doses of benzodiazepine and one other antiepileptic drug (AED), it is called refractory status epilepticus.[4]

SUPER-REFRACTORY STATUS EPILEPTICUS

When seizures continue for more than 24 hours despite giving anesthetic therapy or recurrence of seizures on reduction or withdrawal of anesthetic therapy, it is called super-refractory status epilepticus.[5]

MANAGEMENT (FLOWCHART 1)

Status epilepticus is a medical emergency and treatment should be started as soon as it is known that patient is in status. Treatment of status can be divided in stepwise manner as discussed here.

- Managing the vital parameters
- Management of early status epilepticus (5–30 minutes)
- Management of established status epilepticus (30–60 minutes)
- Management of refractory status epilepticus (1–24 hours)
- Management of super-refractory status epilepticus (>24 hours).

Managing the Vital Parameters

Patients with ongoing seizures are unconscious and are at risk of aspiration as well as cardiorespiratory complications. Their airway, breathing and circulation should be looked at and managed adequately before proceeding further. Supplemental oxygen should be given and if necessary, intubation and mechanical ventilation should be instituted. Intravenous (IV) access should be obtained preferably with a large bore cannula. A rapid neurology screening examination should be done to get any necessary clues regarding diagnosis. Arterial blood gas analysis should be done and samples should be withdrawn for biochemical analysis. Basic investigations which should be done in all patients include blood sugar, electrolytes (sodium, potassium, calcium, magnesium), complete blood count, liver

Manage vital parameters
Identify underlying treatable causes and manage the same
Thiamine and dextrose can be given in alcoholic and malnourished patients

↓

Injection lorazepam 0.1 mg/kg at the rate of 2 mg/min

↓ If seizures continue

Repeat same dose of injection lorazepam

↓ If seizures continue

Either of the following agents can be given
- Injection phenytoin 20 mg/kg at the rate of 50 mg/min
- Injection fosphenytoin 20 mg/kg at the rate of 150 mg/min
- Injection levetiracetam 20–40 mg/kg (1–3 g) over 15 min
- Injection valproate 30 mg/kg at the rate of 10 mg/kg/min
- Injection lacosamide 200–400 mg
- Injection phenobarbitone 20 mg/kg at the rate of 30–50 mg/kg

↓ If seizures continue

Repeat half dose of injection phenytoin/fosphenytoin/phenobarbitone

↓ If seizures continue despite above treatment

It is refractory status epilepticus
Patient will require ICU care, mechanical ventilation and continuous EEG monitoring. Following infusions to be started either alone or in combinations
- Midazolam: 0.2 mg/kg bolus (at the rate of 2 mg/min) every 5 min until the seizure stops up to maximum 2 mg/kg followed by maintenance infusion of 0.1–0.4 mg/kg/h (up to 3 mg/kg/h)
- Propofol: 1–2 mg/kg given over 5 min (at the rate of 10 mg/min) and repeated until the seizure stops followed by maintenance infusion of 2–10 mg/kg/h (maximum 15 mg/kg/h)
- Thiopentone: 3–5 mg/kg at 0.2–0.4 mg/kg/min followed by maintenance dose of 3–5 mg/kg/h

Continued

Continued

Target of treatment is to completely abort seizures and achieve burst suppression pattern on EEG with interburst suppression of at least 10 s for a period of at least 24 h
After 24 h of seizure freedom, gradual tapering of infusions is started under EEG monitoring and drugs are tapered and stopped over next 12–48 h
If seizures recur during tapering then the rate of the infusions is increased to the levels at which seizures are controlled to accomplish above-mentioned target

↓

If seizures continue beyond 24 h despite above treatment
It is super-refractory status epilepticus
Following options either alone or in combination can be tried

- Injection ketamine 2 mg/kg followed by infusion of 1.5–5 mg/kg/h
- Inhalational anesthetics (desflurane/isoflurane)
- Magnesium infusion
- Pyridoxine
- Intravenous immunoglobulins/plasmapheresis
- Hypothermia
- Ketogenic diet
- Surgery
- Electrical and magnetic stimulation

(EEG: electroencephalogram; ICU: intensive care unit)

FLOWCHART 1: Management of status epilepticus.

function tests and kidney function tests. A rapid fingerstick glucose measurement can be obtained till other investigations are pending. In selected patients, brain imaging, AED levels, toxicology screening, cerebrospinal fluid (CSF) studies, autoimmune panel and other necessary investigations can be done simultaneously along with treatment to establish the cause but should not delay the initiation of treatment. Injection thiamine 100 mg and dextrose (50 mL of 50% or 100 mL of 25%) can be given empirically, especially if the patient is alcoholic or malnourished.

Management of Early Status Epilepticus (5–30 Minutes)

Benzodiazepines are the preferred initial drugs used for termination of seizures during first 30 minutes during this gamma-aminobutyric acid (GABA) sensitive phase (GABA receptors which are inhibitory receptors are relatively abundant on neuronal cell surface in early stages of seizures and benzodiazepines act by facilitating GABAergic transmission).[5] Lorazepam is the preferred agent due to its relatively less cardiac and respiratory side effects as well as longer duration of action.[6] It should be given in the dose of 0.1 mg/kg at the rate of 2 mg/min. If the seizure does not terminate in next few minutes, lorazepam can be repeated in the same dose. There is no maximum dose of lorazepam defined that should be given for termination of seizure but care should be taken about potential respiratory and cardiac side effects it can have. Diazepam or midazolam are alternative benzodiazepines that can be given if lorazepam is not available. Meanwhile preparations should be made to load the patient with a nonbenzodiazepine AED. In case seizures stop after giving lorazepam, a long-acting AED has to be given to prevent recurrence of seizures. If patient is already on any AED like levetiracetam or valproate and low serum levels of the same are suspected, loading dose of the same drug can be given. Alternatively loading dose of injection phenytoin or fosphenytoin can be given for preventing recurrence of seizure followed by maintenance therapy.

Management of Established Status Epilepticus (30–60 Minutes)

If seizures continue despite giving two doses of lorazepam, a nonbenzodiazepine AED should be given. This phase of status epilepticus is GABA-resistant phase as there is downregulation of GABA receptors and upregulation of N-methyl-D-aspartate (NMDA) receptors in prolonged seizures.[5] Many agents are available for treatment in this phase.

- *Fosphenytoin/phenytoin*: Loading dose is 20 mg/kg. Fosphenytoin is prodrug which gets converted in phenytoin in the body. It is preferred over phenytoin for few reasons. It is highly water soluble and has less tendency to precipitate during IV administration, it has less tendency to cause local irritation at infusion site hence can be infused at a faster rate (150 mg/min) than phenytoin (50 mg/min). It also has lesser risk of causing hypotension and cardiac arrhythmias as compared to phenytoin making it as safer drug
- *Valproate*: Loading dose is 30 mg/kg given at the rate of 10 mg/kg/min. It is as effective as phenytoin and is preferred agent if the patient has a generalized epilepsy syndrome prior to status
- *Levetiracetam*: Loading dose of 1–3 g (20–40 mg/kg) given over 15 minutes is of comparable efficacy.
- *Phenobarbitone*: Loading dose is 20 mg/kg given at 30–50 mg/min. Though a very effective antiseizure medication, it is less preferred agent nowadays due to slower administration, excessive and prolonged sedation and risk of cardiorespiratory depression. The patient may require intubation to protect airways if phenobarbitone is given after benzodiazepines
- *Lacosamide*: Loading dose is 200–400 mg. It is a newer AED which is coming more and more into practice in patients with status epilepticus, especially in focal seizures. Careful cardiac monitoring is necessary while giving it especially in those with cardiac illness due to the risk of heart blocks.

If the seizure continues despite giving a loading dose of phenytoin or phenobarbitone, half of the initial loading dose can be repeated. At the same time, however, the patient should be considered to be entering the phase of refractory status epilepticus and preparations should be made for giving IV anesthetic agents.

Management of Refractory Status Epilepticus (1–24 Hours)

If the seizure activity continues despite giving initial benzodiazepines and a nonbenzodiazepine drug then it is labeled as refractory status epilepticus. At this point, patient should be put on an infusion of IV anesthetic agents for induction of coma. Such patients require endotracheal intubation and mechanical ventilation in the ICU. Continuous EEG monitoring should also be started. Generally, three agents are available for the induction of coma. Any of the three agents can be started depending on the case scenario.

1. *Midazolam*: It is generally the preferred first-line agent. It is given as 0.2 mg/kg bolus (at the rate of 2 mg/min) every 5 minutes until the seizure stops or a maximum dose of 2 mg/kg is reached. This is followed by continuous maintenance infusion of 0.1–0.4 mg/kg/h which can be gradually increased up to 3 mg/kg/h to maintain seizure freedom. If no control is seen within an hour either propofol or thiopentone infusion is added. An important side effect of midazolam is hypotension but it is less so, than with thiopentone. It has the highest risk of withdrawal seizures on tapering because of tachyphylaxis. Cautious use is advised in those with hepatic and renal impairment
2. *Propofol*: It is another effective drug for induction of coma. The loading dose is 1–2 mg/kg given over 5 minutes (at the rate of 10 mg/min) and repeated until the seizure stops. Following this maintenance infusion is started at the rate of 2–10 mg/kg/h (maximum 15 mg/kg/h). It has a lesser risk of hypotension as compared to other agents and preferred in complex cases with hepatic and renal involvement where pharmacokinetic interactions with other drugs are anticipated. However, its prolonged used beyond 48 hours should be avoided (especially in children) because of the risk of propofol infusion syndrome (PRIS). PRIS is characterized by rhabdomyolysis, metabolic acidosis, cardiac and renal failure. To avoid this complication, dose can be kept below 5 mg/kg/h and duration can be kept below 48 hours especially in the pediatric population and in those on corticosteroids and catecholamine medications. It has lowest risk of hypotension when compared with midazolam and thiopentone

3. *Thiopentone*: Loading dose is 3–5 mg/kg at 0.2–0.4 mg/kg/min followed by maintenance dose of 3–5 mg/kg/h. It has a strong antiepileptic action and is very effective in terminating ongoing seizure hence a preferred agent in severe cases. However, it has a tendency to accumulate in the body resulting in prolonged recovery from anesthesia. Also, multiple pharmacokinetic interactions with other drugs can make it an undesirable agent especially in patients who are on multiple medications. It is also known to cause profound cardiorespiratory depression resulting in severe hypotension requiring vasopressor agents. Thiopentone should be avoided in those with hepatic dysfunction and hypotension.

Goals of the Treatment

The goal of the treatment is to completely stop the seizure and to induce a burst and suppression pattern on EEG for at least 24 hours with interburst suppression lasting at least 10 seconds.[4]

Once therapeutic targets achieved, weaning is gradually started with a reduction in dose every 3 hours with EEG monitoring to look for seizure recurrence. Though there are no guidelines, it is preferable to wean slowly over 12–48 hours as rapid weaning is associated with the risk of seizure recurrence.

If there is recurrence of seizures during weaning or after weaning again the same dose of the agent at which seizures were controlled is restarted and infusion is continued for 24 hours from the occurrence of last seizure.

Management of Super-refractory Status Epilepticus

There are no definite guidelines for management of super-refractory status epilepticus. Treatment options are based mainly on individual case reports and case series. Let us discuss what treatment options are available.

- *Ketamine infusion*: It is an effective and safe drug for treatment of refractory status epilepticus.[7] It has a role in status owing to its NMDA antagonistic actions as there is downregulation of GABA and upregulation of NMDA receptors in prolonged status epilepticus. It is given as loading dose of 2 mg/kg followed by infusion of 1.5–5 mg/kg/h. It has a major advantage of not causing hypotension and at the same time, it has neuroprotective actions due to NMDA antagonism
- *Inhalational anesthetic*: It can be tried if the logistics for the same are available. Desflurane and isoflurane have been used for this purpose in case series. Main advantages are rapid onset of action and high efficacy in stopping seizures.

However, the high risk of complications [hypotension, atelectasis, infection, paralytic ileus, deep venous thrombosis (DVT)] and difficulty in administration makes it a less favorable option[5]

- *Magnesium infusion*: It is useful in the setting of eclampsia, porphyria and mitochondrial disorders. Since it is safe and without significant side effects, it has been tried by many in a noneclampsia setting for control of seizures
- *Pyridoxine*: Though effective in few cases (especially those with the inborn error of pyridoxine metabolism), pyridoxine is given empirically in young children with super-refractory status epilepticus as it is safe and without significant side effect. Its role in adults remains uncertain
- *Immunotherapy*: Immunotherapy in the form of corticosteroids, IV immunoglobulin (IVIg) or plasma exchange is one of the mainstays of therapy in super-refractory cases. Best results are seen in proven cases of autoimmune encephalitis like NMDA receptor encephalitis. However, even though in cases with no apparent immunological cause, immunotherapy can still be given as it is believed that these cryptogenic cases could be due to an immunological cause with yet undiscovered antibodies[8,9]
- *Ketogenic diet*: In many case series and reports, ketogenic diet has shown good results with the complete resolution of seizures where other medical or surgical treatments have failed. Hence it should be tried where feasible
- *Hypothermia*: Reducing temperature up to 31–35°C has been tried for 1–5 days with other methods for control of seizures. It helps in seizure control by decreasing cerebral metabolism, oxygen consumption and cerebral inflammation. Often hypothermia is also employed in the patient with hypoxic brain injury making it a viable option in patients with hypoxic seizures
- *Surgical options*: Emergency neurosurgery can be performed in patients with refractory seizures if a definite seizure focus is identified. A multidisciplinary approach is required for this option. Commonly performed surgeries include lesionectomy, focal resection, lobectomy, hemispherectomy, corpus callosotomy and multiple subpial transections. Few of the above options are palliative rather than curative, aimed at reducing the intensity and frequency of seizures
- *Electrical and magnetic stimulation techniques*: There are isolated reports and case series of the trial of various techniques like vagal nerve stimulation, electroconvulsive therapy, deep brain stimulation and transcranial magnetic stimulation used in conjunction with other methods for control of refractory status with variable results.

MAINTENANCE THERAPY

Maintenance therapy with AEDs is started simultaneously to prevent relapse of status epilepticus. Patients already on AED will require dose escalation or adjustment. In treatment-naïve patients, one of the AEDs which terminated seizure will have to be continued.

COMPLICATIONS OF STATUS EPILEPTICUS

Ongoing seizures can have various ill-effects on the body as mentioned here.[10]

- Seizure-induced cerebral damage
- Cerebral edema, raised intracranial pressure
- Cerebral venous sinus thrombosis
- Hypotension
- Hypertension
- Arrhythmias
- Cardiac arrest
- Respiratory failure
- Hyperpyrexia
- Dehydration
- Electrolyte imbalance
- Acute renal failure
- Acute hepatic failure
- Rhabdomyolysis
- Disseminated intravascular coagulation
- Fractures
- Secondary infections.

PITFALLS IN THE MANAGEMENT OF STATUS EPILEPTICUS

- Misdiagnosis
- Inadequate dosing
- Delay in the institution of second-line drugs
- Delay/failure in starting maintenance therapy
- Failure to detect the underlying/precipitating cause for status epilepticus
- Failure to manage complications of status epilepticus
- Delay in providing cardiorespiratory support, ventilation, vasopressor therapy.

WHAT ARE NORSE AND FIRES?

New-onset refractory status epilepticus (NORSE) is characterized by the onset of prolonged periods of refractory status epilepticus with no identifiable cause in an apparently healthy person. However, various studies have suggested that after extensive evaluation definite etiology can be found in approximately 50% of cases.[8] In those with identified etiology, the most common causes were autoimmune and paraneoplastic encephalitis followed by viral and bacterial central nervous system (CNS) infections. In the cryptogenic cases, it is presumed that yet undiscovered autoimmune or viral encephalitis may be the causative agent. Immunotherapy can prove beneficial in both autoimmune as well as cryptogenic NORSE. A similar illness is described in the pediatric age group called febrile illness-related epilepsy syndrome (FIRES). It is typically seen in the age group of 3–15 years in a previously healthy child and characterized by nonspecific febrile illness often with gastrointestinal or respiratory symptoms followed by the onset of refractory status epilepticus after the fever has subsided. No specific cause or infectious agent is identified and it is postulated that it could be due to an immunological cause and genetic predisposition.[11] Seizures are often refractory to treatment. Use of immunotherapy (IVIg, steroids, plasma exchange), ketogenic diet and hypothermia along with AEDs and anesthetic agents may help in controlling seizures. Children are often left with permanent neurological deficits, intellectual disability and medically refractory seizures.[11]

REFERENCES

1. Guidelines for epidemiologic studies on epilepsy. Commission on Epidemiology and Prognosis, International League Against Epilepsy. Epilepsia. 1993;34:592-6.
2. Trinka E, Cock H, Hesdorffer D, et al. A definition and classification of status epilepticus—report of the ILAE Task Force on Classification of Status Epilepticus. Epilepsia. 2015;56(10):1515-23.
3. Beniczky S, Hirsch LJ, Kaplan PW, et al. Unified EEG terminology and criteria for nonconvulsive status epilepticus. Epilepsia. 2013;54 (Suppl 6):28-9.
4. Rossetti A, Lowenstein D. Management of refractory status epilepticus in adults: still more questions than answers. Lancet Neurol. 2011;10(10):922-30.
5. Shorvon S, Ferlisi M. The treatment of super-refractory status epilepticus: a critical review of available therapies and a clinical treatment protocol. Brain. 2011;134 (Pt 10):2802-18.
6. Treiman DM, Meyers PD, Walton NY, et al. A comparison of four treatments for generalized convulsive status epilepticus. Veterans Affairs Status Epilepticus Cooperative Study Group. N Engl J Med. 1998;339(12):792-8.
7. Gaspard N, Foreman B, Judd LM, et al. Intravenous ketamine for the treatment of refractory status epilepticus: a retrospective multicenter study. Epilepsia. 2013;54(8):1498-503.
8. Gaspard N, Foreman BP, Alvarez V, et al. New-onset refractory status epilepticus. Neurology. 2015;85(18):1604-13.
9. Khawaja AM, DeWolfe JL, Miller DW, et al. New-onset refractory status epilepticus (NORSE)—the potential role for immunotherapy. Epilepsy Behav. 2015;47:17-23.
10. Shorvon S. The management of status epilepticus. J Neurol Neurosurg Psychiatry. 2001;70:1122-7.
11. Fox K, Wells ME, Tennison M, et al. Febrile infection-related epilepsy syndrome (FIRES): a literature review and case study. Neurodiagn J. 2017;57(3):224-33.

14
CHAPTER

When to Start and Stop Antiepileptic Drugs?

Aniruddha Vasant More, Arun Garg, Ashok Panagariya

INTRODUCTION

When a patient presents to physician with the history of a single or multiple seizures, the physician is often faced with multiple challenges right from the diagnosis of seizures, diagnosing correct epilepsy syndrome to the starting of appropriate treatment. It is not uncommon to see a patient who is wrongly treated for many years for seizures when careful history suggests that patient had syncopal attack or nonepileptic events. Once patient is on treatment for seizures, next difficult challenge that the physician has to tackle is regarding discontinuation of the treatment. In this chapter, we will try to answer these questions regarding when to start antiepileptic drugs (AEDs), how long to continue and when to stop the drugs.

First step in starting treatment of epilepsy is to confirm the diagnosis: whether the patient has actually suffered from a seizure? Do not start AED on trial basis—therapeutic trial to confirm the diagnosis. In this way, you may unnecessarily expose patient to AED side effects and, at the same time, you may miss the potentially life-threatening diagnosis like cardiogenic syncope.

CASE

A 65-year-old male got up in the morning and went to toilet to pass urine. When his wife rushed on hearing loud noise, he was on floor, had laceration on his forehead and blood was coming out from his mouth. On asking, he told that while passing urine he felt giddiness, which was possibly followed by sudden fall and loss of consciousness. After consulting physician, he was put on phenytoin sodium 300 mg at bed time. Is he suffering from epilepsy? Is starting AED justified?

Is it Seizure or Syncope?

Before putting any patient on antiepileptic medication, one should confirm whether the episode was truly a seizure or not. Many a time, a patient suffering from syncope is put on antiepileptic medication and he is bound to take it for a pretty long duration unnecessarily. So, how to differentiate syncope from seizure. Table 1 highlights important differences between seizure and syncopal attack.

It is important to note that syncope can be of cardiogenic origin and is characterized by sudden onset and offset, as if you switch on and off an electric device. Cardiogenic events are usually short lasting (for seconds) and recovery is immediate, as if nothing has happened. Other important diagnosis that needs to be differentiated from a true seizure is pseudoseizure or nonepileptic attack disorder (NEAD). Many key points in history and examination will help in differentiating true seizure from pseudoseizure as mentioned in Table 2.

Though side-to-side neck movements and pelvic thrusting indicate possibility of pseudoseizures, these can rarely be seen in hypermotor frontal lobe seizures. Frontal lobe seizures are usually nocturnal and hypermotor and need to be differentiated from parasomnias or sleep-related disorders.

Also go into the details of event before, during and after the ictus. It is the history, which gives you the clues to the diagnosis. All the relevant investigations like magnetic resonance imaging (MRI), electroencephalography (EEG), or cardiac workup including Holter monitoring or even external loop recording may be normal afterwards.

TABLE 1: Difference between seizure and syncope.

Type	Seizure	Syncope
Preictal	It may be in the form of abnormal epigastric sensation, visual, auditory or olfactory aura, psychic feeling. It can happen in any posture	Sinking sensation, impending doom, nausea. Mostly happens when patient is upright. Cardiogenic syncope can happen in any posture
Ictal	Shrill cry, involuntary tonic–clonic movements of limbs, head deviation to either side, incontinence of urine, tongue bite on the side of tongue. Ictal period may last for minutes	Sweating, pallor, occasional tongue bite/incontinence or involuntary movements. Ictal period lasts for seconds
Postictal	Relatively prolonged postictal confusion, amnesia, headache, sleepiness	Immediate recovery, mostly no significant confusion, can recall events that happened prior to ictus

TABLE 2: Difference between true seizure and pseudoseizure.

Characteristics	Seizure	Pseudoseizure
Onset	Often abrupt	Often gradual
Duration	Short (seconds to minutes)	Long (minutes to hours)
Screaming	Usually at onset	During event
Motor manifestations	Tonic posturing followed by jerking	Struggling movements, side-to-side neck movements, pelvic thrusting, patient can lie motionless
Tongue bite	Common, at lateral margins	Uncommon, at tip
Incontinence	Common	Rare
Eyes	Often partially open, upward rolling	Often closed
Offset	Spontaneous	Spontaneous or artificially induced (spraying water)
Injuries	Common	Uncommon
Setting	Can occur anywhere, even when patient is alone	Usually occurs in presence of others, mostly at home

Convulsive movements, incontinence and tongue bite may be rarely seen in neurocardiogenic or cardiogenic syncope (when it is called as convulsive syncope), if blood supply to the brain is compromised for a relatively prolonged period. It is pre-ictal and post-ictal sequence of events, which guides you toward the diagnosis. Also, patient's premorbid status and drug history are important in reaching to a conclusive diagnosis. Any patient who is on diuretics, antihypertensive medications, elderly patients on alpha blockers for prostatic hyperplasia or any other drugs, which have tendency to cause postural hypotension, may suffer from syncopal attack. Syncopal attacks can also be precipitated by activities like bouts of violent coughing (cough syncope) or after micturition (micturition syncope). Young patients are especially prone to have micturition syncope, if they are on any antihistaminic medications or if they had heavy alcohol intake previous night.

APPROACH TO SINGLE SEIZURE

A 20-year-old boy was brought to the emergency with history of generalized tonic-clonic convulsions twice in last 12 hours. On examination, patient was oriented, there was no neurological deficit but bite mark was seen on right side of tongue. On asking, it was revealed that patient did not sleep properly for last 3–4 days because he was preparing for examination. His MRI brain and EEG were normal. Metabolic profile was normal. No history of drug abuse recorded. Should we start AED in this patient?

Is He Suffering from Epilepsy?

When two or more unprovoked seizures occur at interval of more than 24 hours, it is called epilepsy.[1] Seizures occurring in 24 hours, whatever the number is, should be treated as single seizure. The same applies to status epilepticus, if it lasts less than 24 hours. The term unprovoked means absence of temporary or reversible factors lowering threshold for producing seizures (like hypoglycemia, hypocalcemia and alcohol withdrawal).[1]

Can a Patient with Single Seizure be Said to have Epilepsy?

Yes, a single seizure is considered to be equivalent to epilepsy in two situations:

1. If one is diagnosed to have an epilepsy syndrome based on symptomatology or investigations. Best example of this is juvenile myoclonic epilepsy (JME). A patient with JME can present as single seizure but on asking, patient may give the history of spontaneous involuntary jerking of limbs or body since long
2. An elderly patient having a single seizure 1 year after having a stroke or any person with gliotic area or calcification in the brain as a result of previous insult is at a high risk (>60%) of having recurrent seizures and hence can aptly be said to be suffering from epilepsy.

When to Start AED?

The risk of seizure recurrence is around 30–40% after single unprovoked seizure within 1–2 years. If treatment is started immediately after single unprovoked seizure, risk of recurrence is reduced during first 2 years but it does not have any long-term effect on seizure remission. Similarly, risk of treatment-related side effects is also in tune to 20–30%, which may negate the benefit of early treatment.[2]

Similarly, any patient who presents with single provoked seizure with normal neuroimaging and EEG should not be put on AED, as the risk of recurrence is low in such patients, provided desired lifestyle modifications are done. At the same time, conscious effort should be made to find out cause of the seizure and to rule out any epilepsy syndrome or any structural abnormality on neuroimaging. One should also keep in mind the profession of the patient while deciding to start AED. For example, in any patient with profession in which occurrence of seizure can potentially be life threatening (like those working with heavy machineries), threshold to start AED should be low. Serial seizures or those presenting as status are at higher risk of recurrence.

Any person, who has suffered from more than one seizure, 24 hours apart, qualifies to be put on AED, as the risk of seizure recurrence is very high in these patients (57% within 1 year and 73% by 4 years).[2] This applies to all patients whether provoked or not, even with normal MRI and EEG. Single seizure with abnormal MRI showing mass lesion, inflammatory granuloma, vascular pathology, or even gliosis or scar mark from previous insult to the brain mandates AED treatment without delay. Single seizure with normal MRI but abnormal EEG needs judicious analysis and decision. Ideally, such cases should be handled by a neurologist or epileptologist. If EEG is suggestive of primary generalized epilepsy, treatment should be started even after single seizure. Also, single seizure in a patient with mental subnormality or if seizure occurred in sleep, risk of recurrence is high and treatment may be started early after discussing with family.[2]

The Multicentre Study of Early Epilepsy and Single Seizures (MESS) stratified the patients in low, medium and high-risk groups based on the number of seizures occurred so far, associated EEG findings, and neurological abnormality. A score of 0 is given to those who had a single seizure, a score of 1 to those who have thrown two or three seizures, and a score of 2 given to those who have suffered from four or more seizures. Similar one point each is given to patients who are suffering from neurological abnormality and have abnormal EEG. A total score of 1 is associated with medium risk, while a score of 2–4 is associated with a high risk of seizure recurrence.[3]

It has become routine clinical practice to prescribe AED in all patients who have suffered from two or more unprovoked seizures. Certain patients who are suffering from disorders like syndrome of benign partial seizures of childhood may be exempted from this protocol.

Similarly, there is lack of recommendation for patients with minor seizures (simple partial seizures) and for patients with long intervals between seizures. Patients with long intervals between seizures are now put in category of rare seizures and are treated differently (depending on the type of seizure). Hence, if a patient has suffered from only rare complex partial seizures or simple partial seizures, immediate treatment may not be required; but in case of generalized tonic-clonic seizure (GTCS), AED treatment is recommended because of the risk of injury or sudden unexpected death (SUDEP).

ACUTE SYMPTOMATIC SEIZURES

Certain acute medical conditions such as alcohol withdrawal or withdrawal from sedative drugs, metabolic derangements like hyponatremia or hypernatremia, low-calcium levels, acute kidney injury resulting in uremia, and very low or high sugar levels can all result in acute symptomatic seizures in absence of any structural lesion in the brain. Similarly, traumatic brain injury, central nervous system (CNS) infection, or vascular insult (ischemic or hemorrhagic) can also lead to acute symptomatic seizures.

Management goal in all these circumstances should be directed toward identification of the cause and its effective treatment. AEDs, if required, are needed to control seizures in acute phase. Usually, there is no need to continue AED after acute phase is over. Though there are no specific guidelines regarding the duration of therapy in these patients, some recommendations are made as follows:[4]

- Subarachnoid and intracerebral bleed—1 year
- Ischemic stroke and cortical venous sinus thrombosis—1 year
- Mild-to-moderate head injury—only for acute seizure control
- Severe head injury—2 years
- Metabolic and toxic disorders—correction of underlying cause only
- Meningoencephalitis with complete recovery and normal MRI—3 months (if residual focal deficit and/or MRI changes—2 years)
- Cerebral abscess, tuberculoma—2 years
- Parasitic granuloma, if completely resolved with normal MRI—3 months (if persistent/calcified—2 years).

It should be noted that above recommendations are not the rule. Authors prefer to continue AED in all such situations, if follow-up MRI shows persistence of lesion or evidence of gliosis or calcification.

Alcohol withdrawal seizures, also called rum fits, present as single episode of GTCS or brief flurry of multiple seizures within 48 hours of stopping alcohol. These seizures are usually self-limited. Unless recurrent, prolonged, or status, no antiepileptic therapy is required.

Febrile convulsion (FC) is a seizure occurring in children older than 1 month in association with fever (without CNS infection or electrolyte imbalance), no history of previous seizure (without fever), and no recurrence within first 24 hours. Most cases of febrile convulsions are benign, single GTCS lasting for 1–2 minutes (simple FC). Age of onset of FC is between 3 months and 6 years. If FC is focal in onset, associated with Todd's paralysis, has longer duration (10–15 min), or more than one episode occur within 24 hours, it is called complex FC. While the risk of recurrent seizures or epilepsy is low in children with simple FC, risk increases greatly in cases of complex FC in the tune of 8%, 17% and 49% based on one, two, or three associated complicating features, respectively. Besides complex FC and recurrent febrile seizures, positive family history of epilepsy and pre-existing neurodevelopmental abnormalities also predict possibility of later epilepsy. Use of short- or long-term prophylactic AED is not recommended even after two or three isolated febrile convulsions. Treatment is required with benzodiazepines only if seizure lasts for more than 5 minutes or if patient presents with febrile status epilepticus. In such a situation, benzodiazepines can be used to abort the seizure.[5]

Is it Possible to Stop AED?

There are certain epilepsy syndromes where it is advocated to give lifelong AED therapy as the risk of seizure recurrence is found to be very high. While at the other end of spectrum, there are disorders which remit spontaneously and AED can be safely stopped after certain seizure-free interval. Best example of this is benign rolandic epilepsy in which spontaneous remission is seen in almost all the cases. On the other hand, disorders like JME or Jeavons syndrome require lifelong treatment. Diagnosis and knowledge of these syndromes are very important while taking decision to stop AED. It is important to note that only 25% of epilepsy syndromes have a well-defined prognosis. In remaining 75% of epilepsy syndromes, prognosis is intermediate, making decision to withdraw AED tricky. In certain conditions like JME, which requires lifelong treatment, compliance can become an issue along with other social factors like marriage and childbearing in women, which can dissuade patient from taking treatment. These patients of JME can be effectively treated with lower than usual doses of valproate and can be maintained on very small doses of valproate after 2 years of seizure freedom thereby improving compliance issues and reducing risk of fetal malformations in childbearing age.[6] Table 3 shows epilepsy syndromes with well-defined prognosis.[7,8]

In cases of symptomatic epilepsy where prognosis is not well defined, decision is not straight forward and many factors come in to play while deciding to stop AED. There are no clear-cut recommended guidelines regarding AED withdrawal and each case should be individually approached. Following factors are associated with higher risk of seizure relapse after withdrawal and should be considered when a patient is being evaluated for AED withdrawal:[9]

- Longer duration of epilepsy
- Shorter seizure-free interval
- Higher number of seizures before remission
- Presence of structural abnormality on MRI
- Abnormal neurological examination
- Epilepsy onset at adult age
- Focal epilepsy
- Complex febrile seizures in childhood
- Abnormal EEG

TABLE 3: Epilepsy syndromes with well-defined prognosis.

Epilepsy syndrome	Prognosis
Childhood absence epilepsy	75% remission by 30 years of age
Juvenile absence epilepsy	Lifelong treatment
JME	Lifelong treatment
GTCS on awakening	Lifelong treatment
Jeavons syndrome	Lifelong treatment
BECTS	Remits within 3 years of onset
Panayiotopoulos syndrome	Remission within 1–2 years of onset
Idiopathic childhood occipital epilepsy of Gastaut	60% remission within 4 years of onset
Ohtahara syndrome	No spontaneous remission
Early myoclonic encephalopathy	No spontaneous remission
Migrating partial epilepsy of infancy	No spontaneous remission
Severe myoclonic epilepsy of infancy (Dravet syndrome)	No spontaneous remission
Rasmussen encephalitis	No spontaneous remission
Lennox–Gastaut syndrome	No spontaneous remission
Reading epilepsy	No spontaneous remission

(GTCS: generalized tonic–clonic seizure; JME: juvenile myoclonic epilepsy; BECTS: benign partial epilepsy of childhood with centrotemporal spikes)

- Presence of mental retardation
- Multiple seizure types
- Patient on multiple drugs
- History of seizures while on optimal AED dose
- Poor initial response to AED.

Finally, before a decision to withdraw an AED is made, it should be discussed with the patient and family by explaining them the risks and benefits of withdrawing versus continuing them. Many patients may want to continue AED to prevent risk of seizures. This especially becomes important in young females who are planning to conceive or people whose occupation involves hazardous activities like working with heavy machines or driving.

When to Stop Antiepileptic Drug?

Once it is decided that a patient will not require lifelong therapy and decision of stopping the drug is under consideration, next question arises as to how much of seizure-free period is required before stopping the drug. Answer to this question is not straight forward and no clear-cut guidelines exist for the same. In children, at least 2 years of seizure-free interval is necessary before drug withdrawal is attempted.[10] In adults, studies have shown that seizure recurrence was high, if withdrawal was attempted less than 2.5 years after last seizure. Hence in adults, at least 4 years of seizure-free period is recommended before withdrawal is attempted.[7]

How to Stop Antiepileptic Drug?

Once decision is made to stop the AED, next question is how rapidly to stop and if patient is on polytherapy which drug to stop first. Again, no clear-cut guidelines or recommendations are there in these regards. Studies, in children, have shown no difference in relapse rate in children with either rapid withdrawal (4–6 weeks) or slow withdrawal (6–9 months).[11] In adults, no studies are there to address this issue. Hence, many experts believe in tapering slowly over 3–6 months.[9] One important thing that should be kept in mind is that a few AEDs are associated with high risk of withdrawal seizures and these should be tapered very slowly and cautiously. Barbiturate and benzodiazepine group of drugs have highest propensity for causing withdrawal seizures. If patient is on polytherapy then these group of drugs should be the last ones to go off the list. Fortunately, many newer anticonvulsants have very less risk of drug-related withdrawal seizures.

What is the Risk of Recurrence?

Many studies have reported variable risk of recurrence (12–66%) after AED withdrawal.[12] A summary statement given by American Academy of Neurology predicted a chance of successful withdrawal of 69% in children and 61% in adults, if following criteria were met:[13]

- No seizures for 2–5 years
- Only one type of seizure (partial or generalized)
- Neurological examination and IQ are normal
- After successful treatment, EEG is normal.

It was also noted that risk of immediate seizure recurrence increases by two-fold after stopping AED, however, risk after the period of 2 years remained same when compared to those in whom AEDs were continued. This risk of immediate seizures can be minimized by careful selection of patients. Studies in children show that relapse rate varies from 16 to 56%. The risk being highest in the first 6 months which diminishes over time. Maximum relapses (85–90%) were found to occur in first 2 years after withdrawal.[14]

What to do if the Seizures Recur?

If seizures recur during attempted withdrawal or after successful withdrawal, AED therapy should be restarted and continued for the recommended duration before withdrawal is attempted again. However, patient should be re-evaluated to see if he is the candidate suitable for drug withdrawal in future or not. Also, many patients are anxious to know whether they will have medically refractory seizures after relapse and whether they will have same level of seizure freedom after continuation of treatment. Studies have shown that minority of patient (1%) can have medically refractory seizures or poor seizure control after relapse and same should be explained to the patients.[7,15] But majority of them will have same seizure freedom as they had before relapse and studies have shown that AED withdrawal does not change natural history of epilepsy disorder.[9]

CONCLUSION

To conclude, starting and stopping AEDs can be a tricky and difficult situation at times. A rational and individualized approach is recommended in every case for the same.

REFERENCES

1. Camfield P, Camfield C. When is it safe to discontinue AED treatment? Epilepsia. 2008;49 Suppl 9:25-8.
2. Manford M, Cock H. Assessment and investigation of possible epileptic seizures. J Neurol Neurosurg Psychiatry. 2001;70(Suppl 2):ii3–ii8.
3. Rathore C, Paterson R. Stopping antiepileptic drugs in patients with epilepsy in remission: Why, When and How? Neurol India. 2014;62(1):3-8.
4. Strozzi I, Nolan S, Sperling M, et al. Early versus late antiepileptic drug withdrawal for people with epilepsy in remission. Cochrane Database Syst Rev. 2015;(2):CD001902.
5. Tennison M, Greenwood R, Lewis D, et al. Discontinuing antiepileptic drugs in children with epilepsy. A comparison of a six-week and a nine-month taper period. N Engl J Med. 1994;330(20):1407-10.
6. Panagariya A, Sureka R, Sardana V. Juvenile myoclonic epilepsy—an experience from north western India. Acta Neurologica Scandinavica. 2001;104(1):12-6.
7. Schmidt D, Löscher W. Uncontrolled epilepsy following discontinuation of antiepileptic drugs in seizure-free patients: A review of current clinical experience. Acta Neurol Scand. 2005;111(5):291-300.
8. American Academy of Neurology. Practice parameter: A guideline for discontinuing antiepileptic drugs in seizure-free patients—summary statement. Report of the Quality Standards Subcommittee of the American Academy of Neurology. Neurology 1996;47(2):600-2.
9. Incecik F, Mert G, Kiris N, et al. Risk of recurrence after discontinuation of antiepileptic drug therapy in children with epilepsy. J Pediatr Neurosci. 2014;9(2):100-4.
10. Chadwick D, Taylor J, Johnson T. Outcomes after seizure recurrence in people with well-controlled epilepsy and the factors that influence it. The MRC Antiepileptic Drug Withdrawal Group. Epilepsia. 1996;37(11):1043-50.
11. Fisher R, Acevedo C, Arzimanoglou A, et al. ILAE Official Report: A practical clinical definition of epilepsy. Epilepsia. 2014;55(4):475-82.
12. Krumholz A, Wiebe S, Gronseth G, et al. Evidence-based guideline: Management of an unprovoked first seizure in adults: Report of the Guideline Development Subcommittee of the American Academy of Neurology and the American Epilepsy Society. Neurology. 2015;84(16):1705-13.
13. Marson A, Jacoby A, Johnson A, et al. Immediate versus deferred antiepileptic drug treatment for early epilepsy and single seizures: a randomised controlled trial. Lancet. 2005;365(9476):2007-13.
14. Sawhney I, McLauchlan D, Powell H. Management of acute symptomatic seizures: outline of current practice. J Neurol Neurosurg Psychiatry. 2012;83(Suppl 2):A4.1-A4.
15. Patel N, Ram D, Swiderska N, et al. Febrile seizures. BMJ. 2015;351:h4240.

INDEX

Page numbers followed by *f* refer to figure, *fc* refer to flowchart, and *t* refer to table.

C

D

E

J

K

L

M

N

O

P

Q

R

S